GREEN TiO$_2$ AS NANOCARRIERS FOR TARGETING CERVICAL CANCER CELL LINES

GREEN TiO$_2$ AS NANOCARRIERS FOR TARGETING CERVICAL CANCER CELL LINES

MYTHREYI M[1], PATTABI S[1], SENTHILKUMAAR S[2]

[1] DEPARTMENT OF ENVIRONMENTAL SCIENCES, PSG COLLEGE OF ARTS AND SCIENCE, COIMBATORE-641014 TAMIL NADU, INDIA

[2] DEPARTMENT OF CHEMISTRY, PSG COLLEGE OF TECHNLOGY, CIMBATORE- 641004 TAMILNADU, INDIA

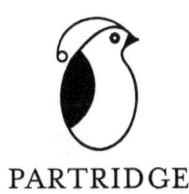

PARTRIDGE

Because of the dynamic nature of the Internet, any web addresses or links contained in this book may have changed since publication and may no longer be valid. The views expressed in this work are solely those of the author and do not necessarily reflect the views of the publisher, and the publisher hereby disclaims any responsibility for them.

Print information available on the last page.

To order additional copies of this book, contact
Partridge India
000 800 10062 62
orders.india@partridgepublishing.com

www.partridgepublishing.com/india

CONTENTS

LIST OF TABLES

LIST OF FIGURES

LIST OF ABBREVIATIONS

ACG	-	Aqueous Chemical Growth
DNA	-	Deoxyribonucleic Acid
DOX	-	Doxorubicin
ED	-	Electro Deposition
EDX	-	Energy – Dispersiv X-ray
FBS	-	Fetal Bovine Serum
FT-IR	-	Fourier Transform Infrared Spectroscopy
GC – MS	-	Gas Chromatography – Mass Spectro metric
HRTEM	-	High resolution transmission electron microscope
JCPDS	-	Joint Committee on Powder Diffraction Microscope
NPS	-	Nanoparticles
P-gp	-	Permeability glycoprotein
PVD	-	Physical Vapor Deposition
QDs	-	Quantum Dots
SAED	-	Selected Area Electron Diffraction Pattern
SEM	-	Scanning Electron Microscope Studies
TEM	-	Transmission Electron Microscope
TiO_2 Ws	-	TiO_2 Whiskers
TIOP	-	Titanium Isopropoxide
UV-VIS	-	Ultraviolet-visible Spectroscopy
VLS	-	Vapor Liquid Solid
XRD	-	X-ray Diffraction

CHAPTER 1

INTRODUCTION

1.1 Nanomaterials

Nanosized particles have been existing on earth since millions of years and are being utilized since thousands of years (Buzea *et al.*, 2007). By definition, a nanostructure is an object that has at least one dimension equal to or smaller than 100 nanometers. There is a wide variety of nanostructures, such as nanoparticles, nonporous, nano rods, nano-wires, nano-ribbons, nano-tubes, and nano-scaffolds. The promising features of these structures are their size dependent properties (Motasim Bellah *et al.*, 2011). Nanotechnology is the art of manipulating materials on atomic or molecular scales especially to build nano scale structures and devices. They may or may not exhibit size related characteristics that differ significantly in comparison to fine or bulk particles. They have gained a whole lot of attention in recent times due to their increasing ability to be synthesized and manipulated, along with their utility in wide areas like electronic, biomedical, pharmaceutical, cosmetics, energy, environmental, catalytic and material applications (Bernd *et al*,. 2007). An estimate for the production of engineered nano materials has been 2000 tons in 2004, which has been predicted to increase 58000 tons by 2020 (Maynard *et al*,.2006)

1.2 Metal oxide nanoparticles

Metal oxide nanoparticles is a special field of materials chemistry that has attracted considerable interest due to the potential technological applications of these compounds in a wide range of fields such as medicine, information technology, catalysis, energy storage and sensing [Corr et al,.2013]. Possess high surface area and high fraction of atoms that is contributing to its various fascinating properties like antimicrobial, magnetic, electronic and catalytic activity. Among the metal oxide nanoparticles, titanium dioxide nanoparticles possess a prominent status and is widely used in air and water purification and in dye-sensitized solar cell due to their oxidation strength, high photo stability and non-toxicity [Monticone et al,. 2000]. Titanium dioxide nanoparticles are being manufactured worldwide in huge amounts for a variety of applications like sunscreen and UV blocking pigments, photo catalyst and electronic storage medium. TiO_2-NPS possess unique physicochemical properties in comparison to their fine particle analogs which may alter their bioactivity. In nanomedicine, intravenous injection is suffient to deliver TiO_2-NPS carriers directly into human body [Shi et al., 2013].

1.3 Nanomaterials in Drug Delivery Studies

Nanotechnology for drug delivery has attracted much attention in recent years. The unique characteristic properties of nanoparticles which are of particular interest for a number of applications are their small size (1-100 nm) and correspondingly large surface to volume ratio, qualitative and quantitative binding properties, high robustness shown by some nanostructure materials. [N.L.Rosi et al., 2005]. Nanoparticles have been used in bio conjugation with peptides, proteins, and DNA and also with some other biological molecules as cellular delivery, labeling, and imaging agents. [Baudhuin et al., 1989; Nel et al., 2006].

In recent years, the convergence between nanotechnology and biology has created the new field of nanobiotechnology. Nanomedicine refers to the usage of nanotechnology in medical applications.

The use of products containing NP is increasing and there is need to understand their toxicity, to fully assess the potential for novel biological uses. Some of the unique properties of nanomaterials have already proven useful in biological applications. For instance, NP are on the same size scale as biological molecules, and so are better able to penetrate tissues and cells and interact with these structures where larger molecules are limited [McNeil *et al.*, 2005]. The surface reactivity of NP makes them easy to modify, either through the addition of drugs or targeting molecules to direct them to specific cell or tissue types [Nel *et al.*, 2006].

Drug delivery is field of research which is gaining the attention of pharmaceutical researchers, medical doctors and industry. Drug delivery can be defined as the process of releasing a bioactive agent at a specific rate and at a specific site

But in the current scenario, Development of techniques that could selectively deliver drugs to the pathological sites is currently one of the most important areas of drug research. The conventional drug delivery techniques have many pharmacy dynamics and pharmacokinetics limitations, such as

- Low efficacy
- Poor solubility
- Low bioavailability
- Quick clearance by Reticulo endothelial system.

This reduced efficacy is due to, Instability of drug inside the cell, Unavailability due to multiple targeting, Chemical properties of delivering molecules, Drug degradation, Changes in signaling pathways with the progression of disease. The Nanoparticle drug delivery system provides increases the aqueous solubility of the drug. It will protect the drug from degradation and also improve the bioavailability of drug. It will provide a targeted delivery of the drug and decrease the toxic side effects of the drug. Nanoparticles offer appropriate form for all routes of administration and also allow rapid formulation development. Nanoparticles applied as drug delivery systems are sub micron sized particles (3-200 nm), devices,

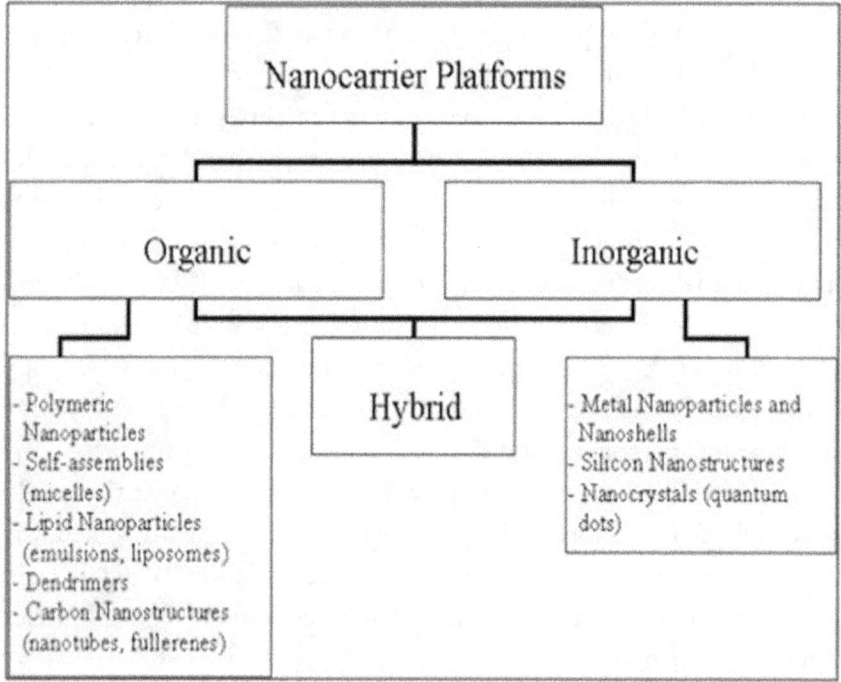

Fig.1 Nanocarrier Platforms

Depending on the method of preparation, the drug is either physically entrapped in or covalently bound to the polymer matrix. Amphiphilic core/shell (polymeric micelles), and or hyper branched macromolecules.

1.4 Nanoparticles in Medicine:

The therapeutic applications of nanoparticles are diverse, ranging from cancer therapeutics, antimicrobial actions, vaccine delivery, gene delivery, Site specific targeting. These nano-particulate systems are very potent against various cancers. Multifunctional NPs with surface functionalized bio molecules are also being synthesized and serve as potential therapeutic agents.

1.5 Cancer

Cancer is a term used for diseases in which abnormal cells divide without control and are able to invade other tissues. Cancer cells can spread to other parts of the body through the blood and lymph systems. Most cancers are named for the organ or type of cell in which they start-for example, cancer beginning in cervix is cervical cancer. Cancer occurs when a cell's gene mutations make the cell unable to correct DNA damage, affect normal cell growth and division. When this happens, cells do not die when they should and new cells form when the body does not need them. The extra cells may form a mass of tissue called a tumor.

There are four key type genes which are responsible for the cell division process.

- ONCOGENES: This genes tells cells when to divide.
- TUMOR SUPPRESSOR GENES: This genes tells cells when not to divide.
- SUICIDE GENES: Control apoptosis and tell the cell to kill itself if something goes wrong.
- DNA-REPAIR GENES: Instruct a cell to repair damaged DNA.

1.5.1 Types of tumors

- Benign tumors- These are not cancerous. They can often be removed, and in, most cases, they do not come back. Cells in benign tumors do not spread to other parts of the body.
- Malignant tumors-These are cancerous. Cells in these tumors can invade nearby tissues and spread to other parts of the body. The spread of cancer from one part of the body to another is called metastasis.

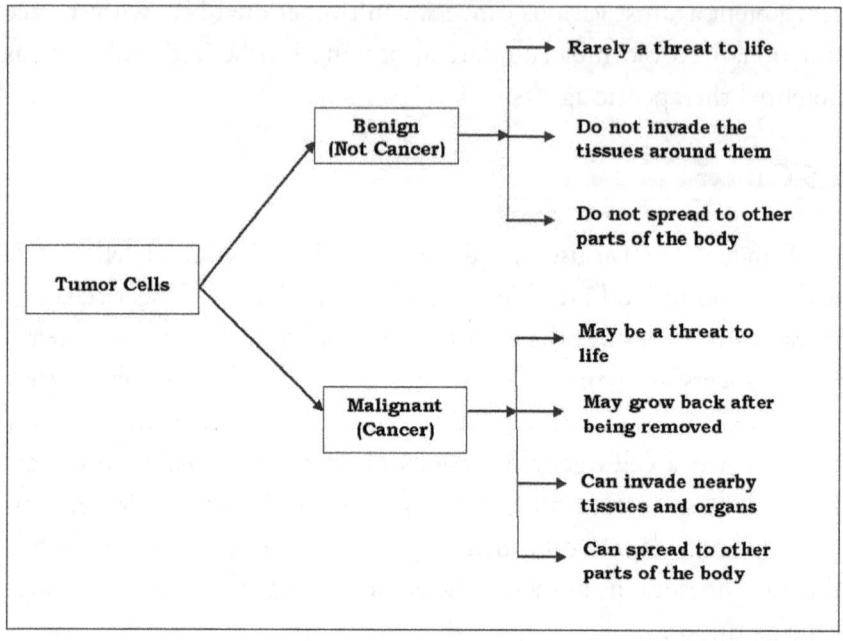

Fig.2 Types of Tumor

1.6 Types of Cancer:

Cancer types can be grouped into broader categories. The main categories include

- **Carcinoma** - That begins in skin or in tissues that line or cover internal organs
- **Sarcoma** - That begins in bone, cartilage, fat, muscle, blood vessels or other connective tissue.
- **Lymphoma and myeloma** - Cancers that begin in the cells of the immune system.
- **Leukemia** - This starts in blood-forming tissue such as the bone marrow and causes large number abnormal blood cells to be produced and enter blood.
- **Central nervous system cancers**- Cancers that begin in the tissues of the brain and spinal cord.

1.7 Requirement of anticancer drug

After administration, an effective anticancer drug should follow two steps. First the drug should reach the desired tumor tissues through the penetration of barriers in the body with minimal loss of their volume or activity in the blood circulation. Second, after reaching the tumor tissue, drugs should have the ability to selectively kill tumor cells without affecting normal cells with a controlled release mechanism of the active form. Nanoparticles seem to have the potential to satisfy both of these requirements for effective drug carrier systems.

1.8 Therapeutic drugs

Commonly used therapeutic drugs that can be encapsulated in nanoparticles are Paclitaxel, Doxorubicin, Carboplatin, Etoposide. Paclitaxel is a mitotic inhibitor used in cancer chemotherapy. Compound is sold under the trademark TAXOL. Paclitaxel is approved in the UK for ovarian, breast and lung cancers.

1.8.1 Carboplatin

Carboplatin is a chemotherapy drug used against some forms of cancer mainly ovarian carcinoma, lung, head and neck cancers.

1.8.2 Etoposide

Etoposide phosphate is an anti-cancer agent. It is available in following brand names like Eposin, Vepesid, and VP-16.

1.8.3 Doxorubicin

Doxorubicin is commonly used in the treatment of a wide range of cancers, including hematological malignancies, many types of carcinoma, soft tissue sarcomas. Leukemia's and Hodgkin's lymphoma, cancers of the bladder, breast, stomach, lung, ovaries, thyroid, soft tissue sarcoma, multiple myeloma, and cervical cancer cells.

1.9 Synthesis of nanoparticles:

Nanoparticles are synthesis using physical and chemical techniques. The physical approach includes techniques such as laser ablation [Z.I Wang *et al.*, 2004], lithography [Vayssieres *et al.,1964*] and high-energy radiation. There are several techniques to synthesize and fabricate nanostructures on different substrates including aqueous chemical growth (ACG) method, vapor-liquid-solid (VLS) method [Wagner *et al.,1964; P.D.Yang et al.*, 2002; X.D.Wang *et al.*, 2005; N.S.Ramgir *et al.*, 2006; J.H.Song *et al.*, 2005; J.H.Park *et al.*, 2006; Q.X.Zhao *et al.*, 2007], metal organic chemical vapor deposition (MOCVD) [W.Lee *et al.*, 2004] and electro deposition (ED) [J.Cembrero *et al.*, 2004; B.Mari *et al.*, 2004].

The chemical synthesis of nanomaterials uses organic solvents and toxic reducing agents. These methods also suffer from other disadvantages, including low yield, high-energy requirements, and a need for difficult and wasteful purifications. A green method for the synthesis of nanoparticles should be distinguished by its use of an appropriate solvent, reducing agent, and stabilizing agents.

1.10 Green Synthesis of Nanoparticles

The need for green synthesis of nanoparticles are essential because of the physical and chemical processes were more expensive and not ecofriendly. So in the search of for cheaper pathways for nanoparticle synthesis, researchers used Microorganisms and then plant extracts for synthesis. Nature has devised various processes for the synthesis of nano- and micro- length scaled inorganic materials which have contributed to the development of relatively new and largely unexplored area of research based on the green synthesis of nanomaterials [B.Mari *et al.*, 2004]. Green synthesis of nanoparticles is a kind of bottom up approach where the main reaction occurring is reduction/oxidation.

The microbial enzymes or the plant phytochemicals with anti oxidant or reducing properties are usually responsible for reduction of metal compounds into their respective nanoparticles.

The three main steps in the preparation of nanoparticles that should be evaluated from a green Chemistry perspective are the choice of the solvent medium used for the synthesis, the choice of an environmentally benign reducing agent and the choice of a non toxic material for the stabilization of the nanoparticles. Most of the synthetic methods reported to date rely heavily on organic solvents. This is mainly due to the hydrophobicity of the capping agents used [Raveendran *et al.*, 2003]. Synthesis using bio-organisms is compatible with the green chemistry principles: the bio organisms are eco-friendly [Li *et al.*, 2007]. Often chemical synthesis methods lead to the presence of some toxic chemical species adsorbed on the surface that may have adverse effects in medical applications [Parashar *et al.*, 2009]. This is not an issue when it comes to biosynthesized nanoparticles as they are eco friendly and biocompatible for pharmaceutical applications.

1.10.1 Use of organisms to synthesize nanoparticles

Biomimetics refers to applying biological principles for materials formation. One of the primary processes in biomimetics involve bioreduction. Initially bacteria were used to synthesize nanoparticles and this was later succeeded with the use of fungi, actinomycetes and more recently plants.

1.10.2 Use of plants to synthesize nanoparticles

The advantage of using plants for the synthesis of nanoparticles is that they are easily available, safe to handle and possess a broad variability of metabolites that may aid in reduction.

A number of plants are being currently investigated for their role in the synthesis of nanoparticles. Gold nanoparticles with a size range of 2- 20 nm have been synthesized using the live Alfa alfa plants [Torresday *et al.*, 2002]. Nanoparticles of silver, nickel, cobalt, zinc and copper have also been synthesized inside the live plants of *Brassica juncea* (Indian mustard), *Medicago sativa* (Alfa alfa) and *Heliantusannus* (Sunflower). Certain plants are known to accumulate higher concentrations of metals compared to others and such plants are termed as hyper accumulators of the plants investigated, *Brassica juncea* had better metal accumulating ability and later assimilating it as nanoparticles. Recently much work has been done with regard to plant assisted reduction of metal nanoparticles and the respective role of phytochemicals. The main Phytochemicals responsible have been identified as terpenoids, flavones, ketones, aldehydes, amides and carboxylic acids in the light of IR spectroscopic studies. While fungi and bacteria require a comparatively longer incubation time for the reduction of metal ions, water soluble phytochemicals do it in a much lesser time. Therefore compared to bacteria and fungi, plants are better candidates for the synthesis of nanoparticles. Taking use of plant tissue culture techniques and downstream processing procedures, it is possible to synthesize metallic as well as oxide nanoparticles on an industrial scale once issues like the metabolic status of the plant etc. are properly addressed.

Previous reports are available for synthesis of TiO_2 nano particle from Annona peel extract [Roopam *et al.*, 2014], *Psidium gujava* [Thirunavukkarasu *et al.*, 2014], [Santhoshkumar *et al.*, 2014], *Catharanthus roseus* leaf extract. We have synthesized the TiO_2 nanoparticle from *Artemesia Pallens* plant extract. *Artemisia pallens*, an aromatic medicinal herb, is cultivated for its fragrant leaves and flowers, which are used in floral decorations, religious offerings, and for the extraction of an essential oil - Davana oil. This oil is mainly used in the flavoring of cakes, pastries, tobacco, and also some costly beverages [Hussain A *et al.*, 2000]. Plants are accredited with anti helmintic, tonic, and antipyretic properties. They are also considered as good fodder. [Ambasta S P *et al.*, 2000]

1.11 Physics and Chemistry of Sol - gel method for preparation of TiO_2 nanoparticles.

Sol-gel method

The sol-gel method is a versatile process used for synthesizing various oxide materials. This synthetic method generally allows control of the texture, the chemical, and the morphological properties of the solid. This method also has several advantages over other methods, such as allowing impregnation or coprecipitation, which can be used to introduce dopants. The major advantages of the sol-gel technique includes molecular scale mixing, high purity of the precursors, and homogeneity of the sol-gel products with a high purity of physical, morphological, chemical properties and using green solvents.

Preparation

In the sol-gel process a molecular precursor in a homogeneous solution undergoes following successive transformations:

i. Hydrolysis of the molecular precursor;
ii. Polymerization via successive bimolecular additions of ions, forming oxo - hydroxyl, or aqua bridges;
iii. Condensation by dehydration;
iv. Nucleation;
v. Growth

Depending on the nature of the molecular precursors, two sol–gel routes are currently used: metal alkoxides in organic solvents or metal salts in aqueous solutions [Senthil Kumar S *et al.*, 2006]. In such media the process involves two steps. The first one consists of in situ formation of alkoxide or alkoxy - complexes. In the second step, these complexes undergo transformation through hydrolysis and polymerization to lead to the oxide. Metal salts are generally used as precursors due to low cost, facility of use and commercial availability.

An overview of sol-gel process steps

The sol-gel process, as the name implies, involves transition from a liquid 'sol' (colloidal solution) into a 'gel' phase [Wright J.D *et.al.*, 2001]. Usually inorganic metal salts or metal organic compounds such as metal alkoxide are used as precursors. A colloidal suspension, or a 'sol' is formed after a series of hydrolysis and condensation reaction of the precursors. Then the sol particles condense into a continuous liquid phase (gel). With further drying and heat treatment, the 'gel' is converted into dense materials. Generally three reactions are used to describe the sol-gel process: hydrolysis, alcohol condensation and water condensation. Because water and alkoxides are immiscible, alcohol is commonly used as co-solvent. Due to the presence of the co-solvent, the sol-gel precursor, alkoxide, mixes well with water to facilitate the hydrolysis.

$$\overset{\displaystyle |}{\underset{\displaystyle |}{-Ti}} - OR + H - OH \;\; \underset{\longleftarrow}{\xrightarrow{\hspace{2cm}}} \;\; \overset{\displaystyle |}{\underset{\displaystyle |}{-Ti}} - OH + R - OH$$

During the hydrolysis reaction, the alkoxide groups (OR) are replaced with hydroxyl group (OH) through the addition of water. Subsequent condensation reaction involving titanol group (Ti-OH) produces titane (Ti-O-Ti) with by-product of water (water condensation) or alcohol (alcohol condensation). As the number of titane group increases, they bridged with each other and a titanium network is formed. Upon drying, the solvents that are trapped in the network are driven off. With further heat treatment at high temperature, the organic residue in the structure is taken out, the interconnected pores collapse.

Hydrolysis and condensation

Although hydrolysis can occur without additional catalyst, it has been observed that with the help of acid or base catalyst the speed and extent of the hydrolysis reaction can be enhanced. Under acid conditions, the alkoxide group is protonated rapidly. As a result, electron density is withdrawn from the titanium atom, making it more electrophilic with partial positive charges. Therefore it's more susceptible to be attacked by the nucleophile, water molecule. Subsequently a penta-coordinated transition state is formed with SN2 type characters, where there is simultaneous attack of the nucleophile and displacement of the leaving group. When the nucleophile attacks the center atom, Ti, it's on the opposite side to the position of the leaving group, R-OH. Finally the transition state decays by breaking of the Ti-OHR bond and ends up with an inversion of titanium configuration as shown in equation. The acid-catalyzed mechanism can be described as following:

$$-Ti - OR + H^+ \underset{\longleftarrow}{\overset{Fast}{\longrightarrow}} -Ti - \underset{H}{O} - R$$

$$-Ti - \underset{H}{O} - R + H - \overset{\cdot\cdot}{OH} \underset{\longleftarrow}{\longrightarrow} \left[\begin{array}{c} R \quad \vee \quad H \\ >O - Ti - O< \\ H \quad | \quad H \end{array} \right]^+ \underset{\longleftarrow}{\longrightarrow} Ti - OH + R - OH$$

Under basic conditions, the hydroxyl anion works as nucleophile and attacks the titanium atom. Again, an SN-2 type mechanism has been proposed in which OH displaces OR group with inversion configuration of the titanium tetrahedron. The mechanism of the base-catalyzed mechanism can be described as following:

$$-Ti - OR + \overset{\cdot\cdot}{OH}^- \underset{\longleftarrow}{\longrightarrow} \left[R - O - Ti - O - H \right]^- \underset{\longleftarrow}{\longrightarrow} R - O - Ti - O - H$$

$$-Ti - OH + RO^-$$

Gelation

In the gelation step, alkoxide gel precursor undergoes polymerization (condensation) reaction with by-product of water or alcohol. Similar to hydrolysis, the condensation reaction is also affected the acid/base catalyst. With the existence of acid catalyst, weakly cross linked polymer is formed and can easily aggregate after drying yielding low-porosity microporous structure. On the contrary, if base catalyst is used, discrete highly branched clusters are formed and lead to a mesoporous structure after gelation.

$$-Ti-OH \ +-Ti \ OH \underset{\text{Hydrolysis}}{\overset{\longrightarrow}{\longleftarrow}} \ -Ti-O-Ti+H-OH$$

$$-Ti-OH \ +-Ti \ R \qquad -Ti-O-Ti+R-OR$$

Ageing

The continuing chemical and physical changes during ageing after gelation are very important. During this process, further cross-links continuous, the gel shrinks as the covalent links replace non-bonded contacts and the pore sizes and pore wall strengths change with the evolution of the gel's structure.

Drying

The gel has a high ratio of water and three dimensional inter-connected pores inside the structure. Before the pore is closed during the densification process, drying, is needed to remove the liquid trapped in the interconnected pores. On the other hand removal of the liquid from the tiny pores causes significant stress resulting from inhomogeneous shrinkage. Therefore the main problem that had to be overcome is cracking due to the large stress in the structure. For small cross sections, such as powder, coating, or fiber, the drying stress is small and can be accommodated by the materials, so no special care is needed to avoid cracking for those sol-gel structures. While for monolithic objects greater than 1 cm, drying stress developed in ambient atmosphere can introduce catastrophic cracking, as a result control of the chemistry of each processing step is essential to prevent cracking during drying.

Densification

Although there are many applications of sol-gel titania prepared and dried at or near room temperature (especially those involving trapping functional organic or biological molecules with the gel pores), heat treatment of the porous gel at high temperature is necessary for the production of dense material from the gel titania. After the high temperature annealing, the pores are eliminated and the density of the sol-gel materials ultimately becomes equivalent. The densification temperature depends considerably on the dimension of the pores, the degree of connection of the pores, and the surface areas in the structure [Hench L. *et.al.*, 1990].

Advantages and limitations of sol-gel method

From the introduction above, the advantages of the sol-gel method become apparent

1. Sol-gel method involves wet chemical synthesis of materials, so the composition of the materials can be tailored at molecular level. As a result, stoichiometrical homogeneous control of the doping is easily achieved.
2. The precursors, such as metal alkoxides, with very high purity are commercially available, which makes it easy to fabricate materials with high quality.

3. It's cost effective because the temperatures required in the process are low, close to room temperature, and no delicate vacuum system is needed.

1.12 Titanium di oxide

Titanium, the world's fourth most abundant metal (exceeded only by aluminum, iron, and magnesium) and the ninth most abundant element (constituting about 0.63% of the Earth's crust), was discovered in 1791 in England by Reverend William Gregor, who recognized the presence of a new element in ilmenite. The element was rediscovered several years later by the German chemist Heinrich Kalporth in rutile ore who named it after Titans, mythological first sons of the goddess Ge (Earth in greek mythology).

Titanium metal is not found unbound to other elements that are present in various igneous rocks and sediments. It occurs primarily in minerals like rutile, ilmenite leucoxene, anatase, brookite, perovskite, and sphene, and it is found in titanates and many iron ores. The metal was also found in meteorites and has been detected in Sun and M-type stars. Rocks brought back from moon during the Apollo 17 mission have 12.1% TiO_2. Titanium is also found in coal, ash, plants, and even in the human body.

Mineral sources are rutile, ilmenite, and leucoxene (a weathering product of ilmenite). 93 to 96% of rutile consists of titanium di oxide, ilmenite may contain between 44% and 70% TiO_2 and leucoxene concentrates may contain up to 90% TiO_2. In addition a high – TiO_2 slag is produced from ilmenite that contains 75-85% TiO_2. About 98% of the world's production is used to make white pigments and only the remaining 2% is used for making titanium metal, welding rod coatings, fluxes and other products.

Ilmenite also called titanic iron ore is a weakly magnetic iron-black or steel-grey mineral found in metamorphic and plutonic rocks. It is used as a source of titanium metal. Kupffer discovered it in 1827 and named it after the Ural Ilmen Mountain (Russia) where it was first found. It is found in primary massive or deposits or as secondary alluvial deposits (sands) that contain heavy minerals. Manganese, magnesium, calcium, chromium, silicon and vanadium are present as impurities. Two-third of the known ilmenite, reserves that can economically be worked up in china, Norway (both having massive deposits), and former Soviet Union (Sands and massive deposits); but the countries with the largest outputs are Australia (sands), Canada (massive ore), and the Republic of South Africa (Sands).

Rutile is the most stable from of titanium di oxide and the major ore of titanium discovered in 1803 by Werner in Spain, probably in Cajuelo, Burgos. Its name is derived from the Latin rutilus, red, in reference, to the deep red color observed in some specimen when the transmitted light is viewed. It is commonly reddish brown but also sometimes yellowish, bluish or violet, being transparent or opaque. Rutile may contain up to 10% iron, and also other impurities such as tantalum, niobium, chromium, vanadium, and tin. It is associated with minerals such as quartz, tourmaline, barite, hematite and silicates. Notable occurrences include Braxil, Seiss, Alps, the USA and some African countries.

Brookite was named in honor of the English mineralogist, H.J.Brooke and was discovered by A.Levy in 1825 at Snowen (Pays de Gales/England). Its crystals are dark brown to greenish black opaque. Crystal forms include the typical tabular to platy crystals with a pseudo hexagonal outline. Associate minerals are anatase, rutile, quartz, feldspar, chalcopyrite, hematite, and sphene. Notable occurrences include those in the USA, Austria, Russia, and Switzerland.

Anatase, earlier called octahedrite, was naned by R.J Hauy, in 1801 from the Greek word, 'anatasis' meaning 'extension' due to its longer vertical axis compared to that of rutile. It is associated with rock crystal, feldspar, and axinite in crevices in granite and mica schist in Dauphine (France) or to the walls of crevices in the gneisses of the Swiss Alps. Besides these polymorphs, two additional high-pressure forms have been synthesized from the rutile phase. These are TiO_2 (II) [Carp O et al., 2003; Hu Y et al., 2003; Simons P Y et al., 1967] with a PbO_2 structure and TiO_2 with a hollandite structure.

Rutile TiO_2 has a tetragonal structure and contains six atoms per unit cell. The TiO_6 octahedron is slightly distorted [Chen X et al., 2007; Thompson et al., 2006; Diebold U et al., 2003]. The rutile phase is stable almost temperatures and pressures up to 60 kbar, where TiO_2 (II) becomes the thermodynamically favorable phase [Norotsky A et al., 1967].

Zhang et al., [Zhang Q et al., 2000] found that anatase and brookite structures transformed to the rutile phase after reaching a certain particle size, with the rutile phase becoming more stable than anatase for particle sizes greater than 14 nm. Once the rutile phase formed, it grew much faster than the anatase. The activity of the rutile phase as a photocatalyst is generally very poor. However, Sclafani et al., [Scalfani A et al.,1990] concluded that the rutile phase can be active or inactive, depending on its preparation conditions.

Anatase TiO_2 also has a tetragonal structure but the distortion of the TiO_6 octahedron is slightly larger for the anatase phase [Linsebigler A et al., 1995; Mo S et al., 1995], Muscat et al., [Muscat J et al., 2002] found that the anatase phase is more stable than the rutile at 0 K, but the energy difference between these two phases is small. The anatase structure is preferred over other polymorphs for solar cell applications because of its higher electron mobility, low dielectric constant and lower density [Carp O et al., 2004]. The increased photo reactivity is because of the slightly higher Fermi level, lower capacity to absorb oxygen and higher degree of hydroxylation in the anatase phase. [Selloni A et al., 2008] reported that the reactivity of (001) facets is greater than that of (101) facets in anatase crystal. Synthesized uniform anatase crystals containing 47% (001) facets using hydrofluoric acid as a morphology controlling agent.

Brookite: Brookite TiO_2 belongs to the orthorhombic crystal system. Its unit cell is composed of 8 formula units of TiO_2 and is formed by edge-sharing TiO_6 octahedral. It is more complicated, has a larger cell volume and is also the least dense of the three forms and is not often used for experimental investigations [Thompson T L et al., 2006]. Heat treatment has a vital role in the synthesis of particles, affecting morphology, crystallinity and porosity, and causing a decline in surface area, loss of surface hydroxyl groups and inducing phase transformation. At high temperatures (400°C and above) the removal of organic materials takes place. The surface area of TiO_2 decreases with calcinations time and heating rate because of the collapse of pores in the TiO_2 powder caused by the transformation of amorphous TiO_2 to the anatase phase. Slow heating rates provide relatively mild conditions for phase transformation [You X *et al.*, 2005] Hu *et al.*, reported that TiO_2 normally undergoes an anatase-to-rutile phase transformation in the range from 600–700°C. The transformation was also affected by factors such as preparation conditions, precursors, impurities, oxygen vacancies and the primary particle size of the anatase phase. [Hu Y *et al.*, 2003].

Hence with the above background information the present study is aimed with the following objectives.

1.13 Research objectives

- ❖ Extraction of water soluble organics from the *Artemissia pallens* plant through distillation process
- ❖ Characterization of the solvent extracted from *Artemisia pallens* plant
- ❖ Identification of the chemical components of the extract
- ❖ Synthesizing titanium dioxide nanoparticles using the green solvent extracted from the *Artemisia pallens* instead of commercial alcohol
- ❖ Studying the structural and morphological characteristics of the as synthesized titanium dioxide nano particles
- ❖ Doping of titanium dioxide nano particles with commercially available anti cancer drug Doxorubicin and studying the characteristics of Doxorubicin doped TiO_2 before and after retention time
- ❖ Cytotoxicity studies are carried out for control, TiO_2 and Doxorubicin doped TiO_2 in cervical cancer cells

CHAPTER 2

---◆●◆---

REVIEW OF LITERATURE

2.1 TiO$_2$ nanoparticles

A significant amount of research on TiO$_2$ has been performed over the last five decades and a number of reviews on various aspects of TiO$_2$ have been published [Fujishima A *et al.*, 2000; Carp O *et al.*, 2004; Mor G K *et al.*, 2006; Chen X *et al.*, 2007; Thompson T L *et al.*, 2006; Diebold U *et al.*, 2003; Linsebigler A L *et al.*, 1995]. Nanoparticles have been prepared by many methods such as Langmuir-Blodgett films, vesicles Youn *et al.*, [H.C. Youn *et al.*, 1998; M. Toba *et al.*, 1994] and reverse micro - emulsions Fendler *et al.*, [K.C. Yi *et al.*, 1990]. The chemical and physical properties exhibited by these materials depend, among others, on both the composition and the degree of homogeneity.

2.2 Synthesis of nanoparticles

Therefore, different synthesis strategies have been developed Toba *et al.*, [M. Toba *et al.*, 1994, X. Gao *et al.*, 1999]. Such as co-precipitation, flame-hydrolysis, impregnation, chemical-vapour deposition, etc. The sol-gel route has demonstrated a high potential for controlling the bulk and surface properties of the oxides [Ward *et al.,1995;* Liu *et al.*, 1994; Schraml-Marth *et al.*, 1992]. Depending on the drying conditions the binary oxides could be obtained as aerogels, either by supercritical drying [Pajonk *et al.*, 1991], [Dusi *et al.*, 1999], or by silanization of the material previously to a conventional drying [Sotelo *et al.*, 1999]. Additionally, non-hydrolytic sol-gel routes have been also reported in the literature. [Hay *et al.*, 1998, Venkatachalam *et al.*, 2007; Sharmila devi *et al.*, 2014; Rayes caranado *et al.*, Kiyoshi kane *et al.*, 2004; Bessekhouad *et al.*, 2003; Zhou, *et al.*, 2006; Byun *et al.*, 2000]

2.3 Green synthesis of nanoparticles

Conventionally, nanoparticles have been mostly synthesized by physical and chemical methods, which are potentially hazardous, requiring high energy along with difficulty in separation process [Taleb *et al.*, 1997; Rodriguez – Sanchez *et al.*, 2000; Krishna *et al.*, 2009; Tripathi *et al.*, 2010; Saxena *et al.*, 2010] Biosynthesis involves using an environment-friendlygreen chemistry based approach that employs unicellular and multi cellular biological entities such as actinomycetes [Ahmad *et al.*, 2003; Sastry *et al.*, 2003], bacteria [Roh,.*et al.*, 2001; Lengke *et al.*, 2006; Nair *et al.*, 2002; Joerger *et al.*, 2001; Husseiny *et al.*, 2007; Mukherjee *et al.*, 2001], fungus [Ahmad *et al.*, 2003; Ahmad. A *et al.*, 2005; Kuber *et al.*, 2006], plants [Philip.D *et al.*, 2010; Kumar *et al.*, 2011], viruses [Lee *et al.*, 2002; Merzlyak *et al.*, 2006], and yeast [Dameron *et al.*, 1989; Kowshik *et al.*, 2003; Gericke *et al.*, 2006]. Due to the diversity of plants, nanoparticles synthesis from plants has known an interesting subject across the world as different plant species are being rapidly investigated and used in nanoparticles synthesis [S. Baker *et al.*, 2013].

Platinum nanoparticles were synthesized using leaf extract of *Diopyros kaki*. The synthesized platinum nanoparticles were characterized resulting in 2 to 12nm in size FTIR analysis revealed that the formation of platinum nanoparticles was due to the biomolecules present in the extract but not an enzyme mediated process [Song J.Y *et al.*, 2010]. The synthesis of iron and silver nanoparticles were studied using the aqueous bran extract of *Sorghum*. The synthesized silver nanoparticles were crystalline in nature with an average diameter of 10nm in size and face centered cubic shaped whereas the iron nanoparticles were amorphous in nature with a 50nm average diameter size [Njagi C.E *et al.*, 2011]. Biological synthesis of gold nanoparticles using *Nyctanthe sarbortristis* ethanolic flower extract was evaluated resulting in synthesis of spherical shaped gold nanoparticles with size 19.8 ± 5.0 nm[Das R.K,. *et al.*, 2011]. The photosynthesis of titanium dioxide nanoparticles using *Nyctanthes* leaf extract resulted in formation of titanium dioxide nanoparticles which was analyzed by SEM and PSA resulting in the size ranging from 100 to 150nm [Sundrarajan M,. *et al.*, 2011]. The synthesis of selenium (SE-protein) composites using *Capsicum annuum*L. extract resulted with the increased concentration of *Capsicum annuum* low pH increases the SE-protein composites of the shell [Sundrarajan M *et al.*, 2007]. Similarly synthesis of zinc oxide using procera latex revealed zinc nanoparticles which was analyzed by TEM and SEM that revealed the particles size ranging 5-40 nm and spherical shaped respectively [Singh P.R *et al.*, 2011]. The aqueous leaves extract of the *Sorbusaucuparia* were used as reducing agent for the synthesis of silver and gold nanoparticles. The formation of silver and gold nanoparticles were characterized by electron microscopy (TEM), UV-Vis spectroscopy, X-diffraction (XRD), energy dispersive X-ray (EDX) and Fourier transform in-fared spectroscopy (FTIR). The concentration of residual silver and gold ions were measured by Inductively Coupled Plasma (ICP) spectroscopy. The synthesized nanoparticles were spherical, triangular and hexagonal in shape with an average size of 16 and 18nm for silver and gold respectively [Dubey S.P *et al.*, 2010]. Similar study conferring green synthesis of silver nanoparticles using weed Argemone mexicana leaf extract was reported which was monitored by UV spectroscopy, FTIR, XRD and SEM. X-ray diffraction and characterized by SEM analysis resulted in the average particlesize of 30 nm[Singh A *et al.*, 2010]. Plant mediated silver nanoparticles using the sea weed Padinatetrastromatica leaf extract upon evaluation resulted in silver nanoparticles formation which was confirmed by analytical techniques. Fourier Transform Infraspectroscopy analysis revealed that bimolecular compounds were capped with nano-silver are responsible for reduction of silver ions [Jegadeeswaran P *et al.*, 2010.]

2.4 Green Synthesis of TiO$_2$ Nanoparticles Using Plant Extract

1. *Nyctanthes Arbor-tristis*

Sundrarajan and Gowri, (2011) [Sundrarajan M. *et al.*, 2011] synthesized TiO$_2$ NPS by the reaction between titaniumtetraisoproxide and ethanolic leaf extract of nyctanthes arbor-tristis under stirring at 50°C for4 hours. Then calcinated it at 500°C. TiO$_2$ NPS where characterized by XRD, SEM and particle size analyser. XRD revealed that the average grain size formed by Bio synthesis wasnear 100nm. SEM study demonstrated that average size of synthesis TiO$_2$ NPS were 100-150nm and morphology was spherical.

2. *Jatrophacurcas L*

[Hudlikar*et al.*,2012] explained that TiO$_2$ NPS produced by the reaction between latex of Jatrophacurcas L and TiO(OH)$_2$. XRD & TEM revealed that the size of synthesized TiO$_2$ NPs were 100-200nm. FTIR spectra of latex capped TiO$_2$ NPS showed the presence of capping / stabilizing agent like protein / peptide material which also prevent the nanoparticles from agglomerization.

3. *Ecliptaprostrata*

[Rajakumar *et al.*, 2012] synthesized TiO$_2$ NPS using aqueous extracts of Ecliptaprostrata leave as bio templating agent. The precursor that has been used was of TiO (OH)$_2$. The obtained TiO$_2$ NPS were spherical in shape and their size ranged from 36 nm to 68 nm. And the calculated average size of synthesized TiO$_2$ NPS was 49.5 nm.

4. Paddy (Orizasativam)

Ramimoghadam *et al.*, 2014 synthesized TiO$_2$ NPS using rice straw powder as biotemplate with titanium tetraisopropoxide aqueous solution and acetic acid. The above mentioned solution was heated at 80°C to form gel. The obtained gel was dried at 80°C and Calcined at 500°C for 5 hours. The average size of synthesized TiO_2 NPS was 10-20nm.

5. Psidiumguajava

Kumar *et al.*, 2014 synthesized TiO_2 NPS using aqueous extract of *Psidiumguajava* leaf and $TiO(OH)_2$ used as precursor. To synthesize TiO_2 NPS 20 ml aqueous extract of *P.Guajava* was added into 80 ml of $TiO(OH)_2$ at room temperature under stirred condition for 24 hours. The XRD pattern of the synthesized TiO_2 NPS showed the presence of both anatase(110) and rutile (111) crystallographic structure. The calculated average size of plant synthesized TiO_2 NPS was 32.58 nm.

6. Neem

An eco-friendly method for the green synthesis of TiO_2 NPS using ethanolic extract of neem as biotemplate was developed by Shilpa Hiremath *et al.*, 2014. For synthesis of TiO_2 NPS, titanium tetraisopropoxide was used as the precursor. The XRD pattern of synthesized TiO_2 revealed that obtained TiO_2 formed anatase crystal mainly and calculated average diameter of the grain was 18 nm. From the particle size distribution of the synthesized TiO_2, it was obtained that 90% of the particle existed within 100 nm. size.

7. Aloe Vera

Nithya *et al.*, 2013 bio synthesized TiO_2 NPs using aqueous extract of Aloe Vera gel as biotemplate. $TiO(OH)_2$ was used as the precursor. For synthesis of TiO_2 NPS, 100 ml $TiO(OH)_2$ and 5ml and 20 ml of aq. extract of aloe vera gel were stirred for 24hrs. The XRD pattern of synthesized TiO_2 NPs showed that the crystal structure was predominantly anatase and calculated average partical size was about 11nm. Atomic force microscopy image in two dimensional view of obtained TiO_2 revealed the size of the synthesized partical was between 80-90nm.

8. *OcimumbasilicumL*.var.purpurascensBenth.- LAMIACEAE

TiO$_2$ NPs were prepared by salam and siraraj *et al.*, 2014 from the aqueous leaf extract of Ocimum basilicumL. var. Benth.- LAMAIACEAE. The precursor used was titanium (iv) isopropoxide. To synthesized the TiO$_2$ NPS, the crude aqueous leaf extract and the ethanolic solution of the precursor were taken in the ratio 1:9 and it was subjected to stirring for 4hrs at 50°C after washing and centrifugation the obtained TiO$_2$ NPs which was calcined at 500°C for three hours. The particle size of the synthesized TiO$_2$ NPs was found 6.97nm as per scherrer equation. TEM image revealed that the morphology of obtained TiO$_2$ NPs was hexagonal and average particle size was 50nm.

9. *Albiziasaman*

Subhashini and Vallinachiyar *et al.*, 2014 synthesized TiO$_2$ NPs via green root using aqueous extract of AlbiziaSaman leaf. TiO$_2$ was used as a precursor. For synthesis of TiO$_2$ nanoparticles, aqueous solution of TiO$_2$ was added drop wise in to the aqueous leaf extract with stirring at 50°C. The XRD pattern revealed the particle size of obtained TiO$_2$ NPs was 41nm and with anatase crystal of TiO$_2$ predominately.

10. *CassiaAuriculata*

Valli and Geethat *et al.*, 2015 synthesized TiO$_2$ NPs using ethanolic extract of Cassia Auriculata leaf. The precursor that have been used was Titanium(iv) isopropoxide for the synthesis of TiO$_2$ NPs 50 ml ethanolic leaves extract were added to 4ml titanium tetra isopropoxide under stirring at 50°C. FESEM revealed that the average particle size of obtained TiO$_2$ NPs was from 38-44.2 nm.

11. Orange (citrus sinensir L)

Rao *et al.*, 2015 synthesized TiO_2 NPs using aqueous extract of orange pill as reducing agent. Titanium(iv) isopropoxide solution drop wise under constant stirring at pH 7 for 3 hrs. The obtained TiO_2 NPs calcined at 600°C for 3hrs for obtaining rutile phase. The average crystallite size of obtained TiO_2 NPS was calculated as 19nm using Debye scherrer's Formula. The average particle size of synthesized TiO_2 NPs was obtained by particle size analyser as 24nm.

12. *CalotropisGiganta*

Marimuthu *et al.*, 2013 synthesized TiO_2 NPs using aqueous extract of *c.giganta* flower. $TiO(OH)_2$ was used as precursor. For synthesis of TiO_2 NPs, aqueous plant extract was added with precursor with constant magnetically stirred for 6 hrs. Then the mixture was subjected to ultra sonication for 30 minutes to separate out agglomerates formed. SEM micrographs of obtained TiO_2 NPs showed the aggregated, spherical in shape with average size between 160-220 nm.

With the help of this literature knowledge we developed a novel method to synthesis titanium di oxide using *Artemisia pallens* plant extract. This extract itself act as reducing and capping agent and we have not used any other external alcoholic solvent in our synthesis method.

2.5 Nanoparticles of Biomedical Importance

Due to their unique physical, chemical and electronic characteristics, nanoscale engineered particles find broad application for energy, environmental, and, more recently, biomedical applications [Aznar E *et al.*, 2015; CheE *et al.*, 2015; Hughes GA *et al.*, 2015; Chung C *et al.*, 2013; Dykman *et al.*, 2012]. There are some reports that claim the nanoscale form of metallic gold was used for medicinal purposes as early as 2500 B.C. by civilizations in India, China, and Egypt [Chaudhary A *et al.*, 2007; Pal D *et al.*, 2014]. However, recently there has been a mushrooming of applications in the biomedical arena due to advances in the science of synthesis and characterization. Tunable geometric, optical, and surface properties of organic and inorganic nanomaterials enables engineering for a number of applications, such as drug delivery, controlled release, deep tissue imaging and sensing of cellular behavior.

2.6 Nanopaeticles for Drug Delivery

Nanotechnology-based novel drug delivery approaches address issues associated with the current pharmaceutical approach by enhancing shelf-life and acceptability either by uptake efficacy or patient compliance [De Villiers *et al.*, 2008; FarokhzadOC 2009; *et al.*, Sahoo SK *et al.*, 2003]. Nanoparticles can be delivered by various entry routes, including oral administration [GelperinaS *et al.*, 2005; Pridgen EM *et al.*, 2015], vaccination [Smith JD *et al.*, 2015] and aerosol-based drug delivery [Dames P *et al.*, 2007; Beck-Broichsitter M, *et al.*, 2012; Chattopadhyay *et al.*, 2013] depending on the therapeutic requirement. The selection of the drug administration approach is based principally on the target localization, drug retention time, physiological barriers and pathobiology of the target disease [Labhasetwar V *et al.*, 2005]. Despite the potential risk of spreading infectious diseases, the invasive technique of vaccination is still an important instrument to deliver drugs to animals and humans. For instance, Jung *et al.*, established a methodology for topical vaccination using nanosized liposomes in the hair follicle. Liposomes penetrate deeper into hair follicles than a standard formulation, leading to an increased trans-follicular drug uptake. The uptake of liposome further depends on surface charge [ChattopadhyayS *et al.*, 2013; Labhasetwar V *et al.*, 2005; Jung S *et al.*, 2009; Chadha TS *et al.*, 2012]. Alternative, non-invasive approaches, such as nasal-based mucosal and oral administration of drugs, has become more popular but widespread use is constrained due to drug insolubility problems [Csaba N *et al.*, 2009]. Another noninvasive approach of pulmonary drug delivery based on aerosol science and technology is used for the treatment of respiratory disorders such as asthma, cystic fibrosis, respiratory infection and lung cancer [O'Riordan TG *et al.*, 2005; Dinwiddie R *et al.*, 2005; Hagerman JK *et al.*, 2006; Rao R *et al.*, 2003].

2.7 TiO_2 as nanocarrier for cancer treatment

As a suitable candidate for drug delivery system, Titanium Dioxide (TiO_2) or titania, a metal oxide semiconductor, attracted emerging attention, mostly due to its photo catalytic activity and chemical stability as well as low-cost and low-toxicity [Yin ZF *et al.*, 2013; Linsebigler AL *et al.*, 1995]. Many TiO_2 nanostructures, including TiO_2 NPs, TiO_2 nanotubes, TiO_2 matrices, as well as TiO_2 capsules and TiO_2 whiskers (TiO_2 Ws), have been used as drug delivery systems for different anti-cancer drugs, such as Daunorubicin (DNR), Temozolomide (TMZ), Gambogic Acid (GA), Doxorubicin (DOX), cisplatin and valproic acid [Li QN *et al.*, 2009; Lopez T *et al.*, 2006].

CHAPTER 3

MATERIALS AND METHODS

3.1 Materials

The precursor, Titanium-iso-propoxide obtained from Alfa Aesar and used as such without any further purification. The drug, Dox obtained from Khandelwal Laboratories Ltd., of molecular formula $C_{27}H_{29}NO_{11}$ and molecular weight of 543.525 g/mol. The water used in our research is of doubly distilled quality. All the glassware's used are Schott-Duran and Borosil glass quality. Bio-Extract is prepared instantly and used immediately, in order to avoid de-nature.

3.2 Collection and Preparation of *Artemisia pallens* extract

The fresh *Artemisia pallens* plant of Family: Asteraceae Genus: Artemisia Species: *A.Pallens* collected from the local flower market, Coimbatore, Tamil Nadu, India.

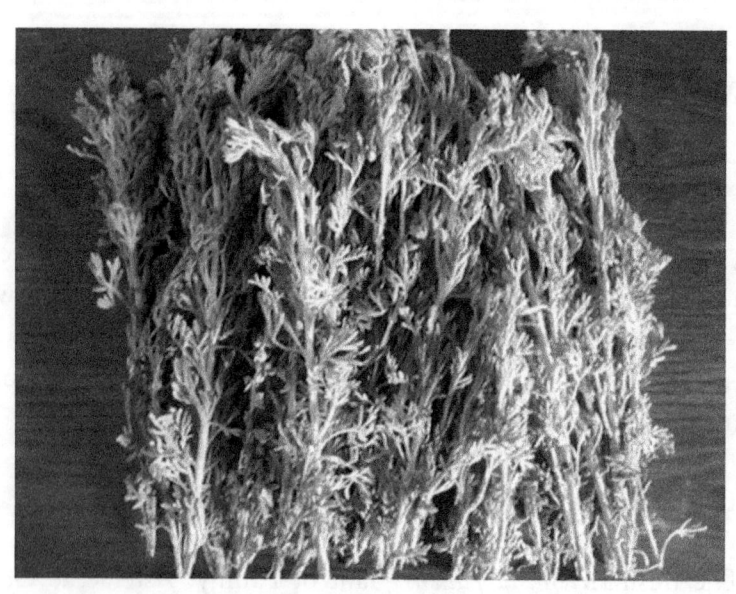

Fig.3 *Artemisia pallens plant*

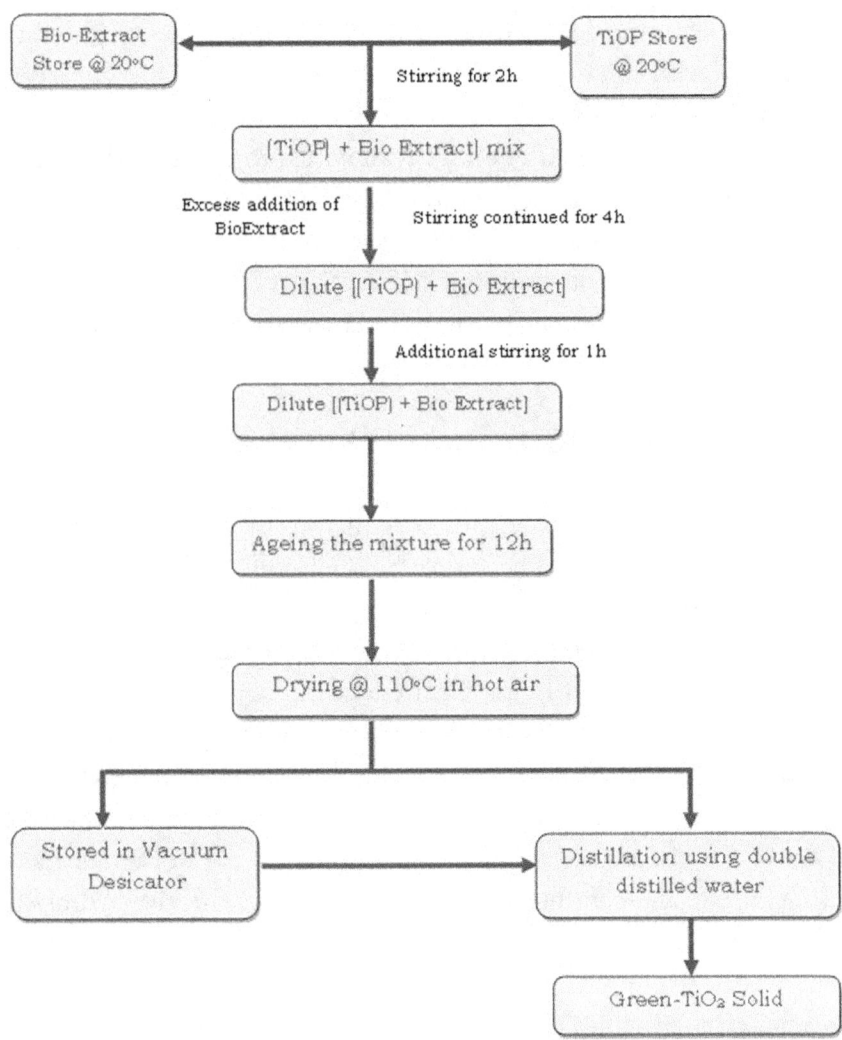

Fig.4 Scheme of Bio-Extraction

The scheme of bio-extraction is shown in Fig.4 It was thoroughly washed with tap water to remove the soil and dirt. The plant leaf along with stem was cut into small pieces and made into slurry using mixer grinder using doubly distilled water. The slurry was subjected to distillation with 150 ml of double distilled water in a soxhlet appratus. The condensed liquids, called bio-extract, were collected in an air-tight round bottomed flask. The residue is subjected to re-distillation using doubly distilled water to ensure possible extraction of the bio-materials. In order to understand the chemical composition, the bio-extract was subjected to GC-MS analysis (GCMS-QP2010 PLUS Shimadzu) and FT-IR spectrum analysis. This bio-extract was used as a solvent for the synthesis of nano TiO_2.

3.3 Synthesis of Nano TiO_2 using Bio-Extract

Titanium iso propoxide is used as the precursor for the synthesis of TiO_2 nano particles. The simple Sol-Gel route is followed for the synthesis, using the bio-extract obtained from Artemisia pallens as solvent for the effective hydrolysis. A schematic scheme of preparation of TiO_2 is presented in figure 5. Twenty milliliters of the bio-extract is added to the 500ml round bottom flask containing 7g of Titanium isopropoxide. The mixture is stirred in a magnetic stirrer, (REMI 1 ml Magnetic Shaker) at 100rpm at room temperature for 2h. After 2h, 25ml of the bio-extract is added dropwise to the round bottom flask using burette and continued the stirring for 4h for effective hydrolysis of the precursor, the mixture is stirred for further 1h and aged for 12h. The aged mixture is then transferred to a 50ml glass beaker and kept in a hot air oven at 100°C, for 3h. The dried solid is then transferred to silica crucible and calcined at 500°C for 1h in a temperature controlled muffle furnace (Technico). After 1h, the contents in the silica crucible is cooled to room temperature and stored in a vaccum desicator. The solid, obtained is labeled as Green-TiO_2 and subjected to characterization using standard procedures.

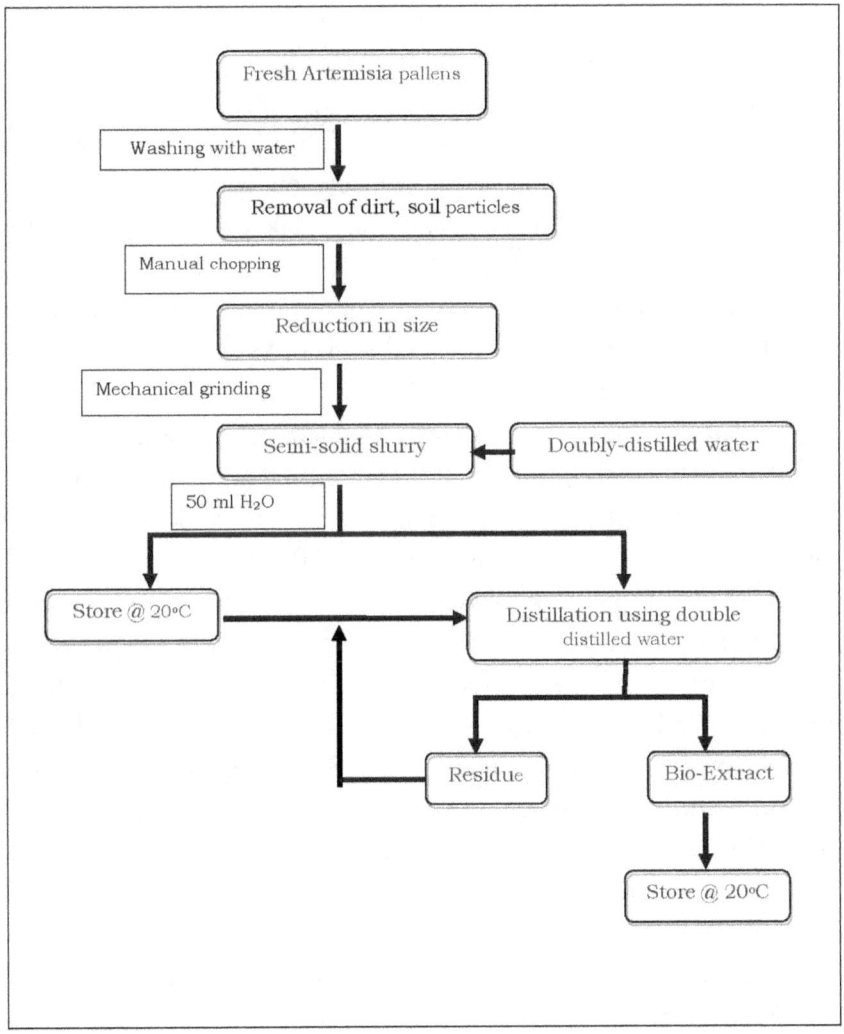

Fig.5 Scheme of Sol-gel-TiO₂

3.4 Drug Encapsulation over Green-TiO$_2$ nanoparticle a Drug – Carrier

In order to optimize the drug encapsulation over Green-TiO$_2$, we fixed the concentration of drug (10mg) and Green- TiO$_2$ (50mg) by varying the pH of the solution and time.

In a typical experiment, the drug, DoX, 10 mg is dissolved in 5ml of the distilled water in 25ml conical flask. This slurry is further diluted with 45ml of double distilled water. The content in the conical flask is equilibrated for 1h in a mechanical rotary shaker. After 1h, the flask from shaker and the pH of the DoX slurry was noted, also complete wavelength scanning made using UV-Vis absorption Spectrophotometer. The pH of the DoX Slurry was found to be 6.0 and shows maximum absorption at 483 nm.

The fifty millilitres of the slurry is divided into four equal volumes in different 100ml conical flask and are adjusted to desired pH values, using the acidic/basic buffer solution. All the four conical flasks were equilibrated until to the desired pH values, 3.0, 6.0, 8.0 and 10.0. After equilibration the supernatant was analysed by UV-Vis spectrophotometer and also pH.

Fifty milligram of Green-TiO$_2$ is added to the 50ml double distilled water in 100ml conical flask. The contents in the conical flask were adjusted to the desired pH values, 3.0, 6.0, 8.0 and 10.0 and equilibrated in a mechanical rotary shaker. After equilibration, the supernatant was discarded and the contents were dried in an hot-air oven at 60°C for 6h.

The pH equilibrated Green-TiO$_2$ was mixed with the pH equilibrated DoX solution in 100ml conical flask. Thus the contents in the conical flask were subjected to equilibration in a mechanical shaker machine at 120 rpm. The conical flasks were withdrawn from the shaker at pre-determined time intervals 6, 12 and 18h.

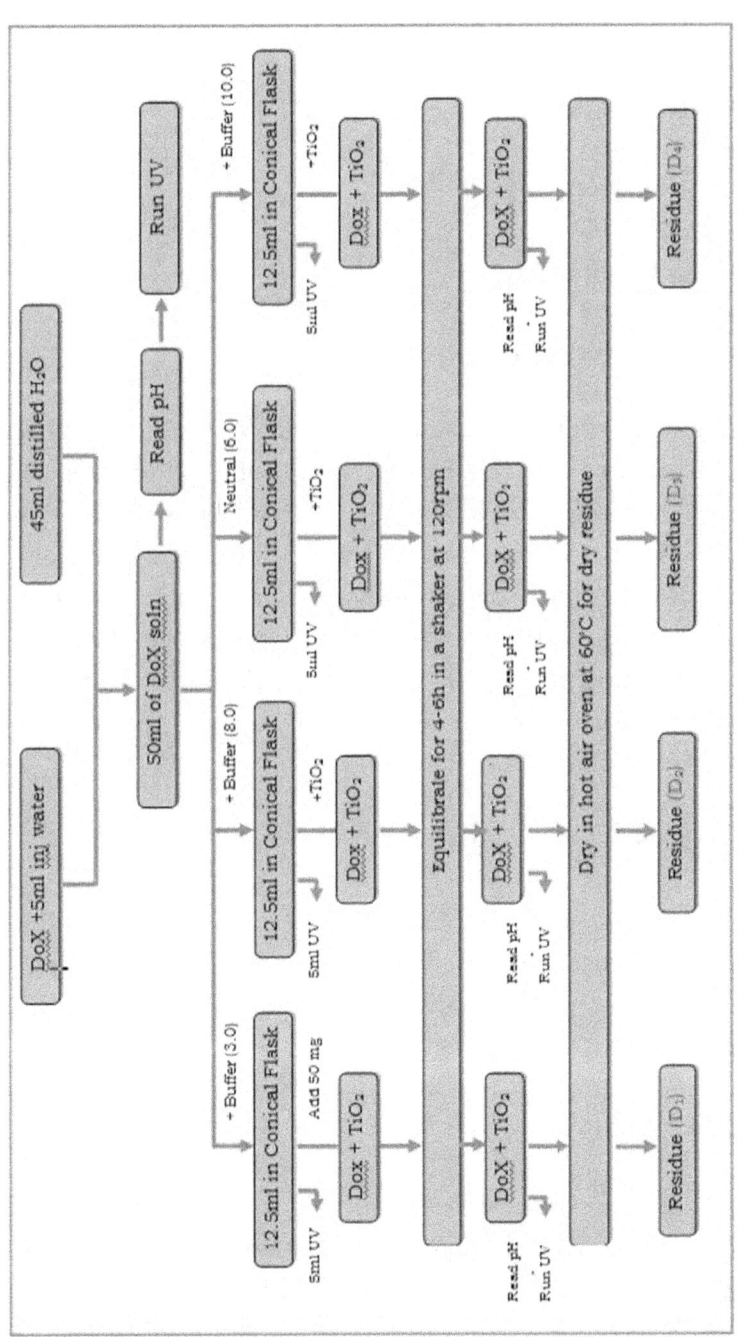

Fig.6 Scheme of Drug Encapsulation over Green-TiO$_2$

35

The supernatant solution was separated by membrane filtration and subjected to UV-Vis analysis. The solid, DoX encapsulated Green-TiO_2 was further activated in a hot-air oven at $60°C$ for 2h. The drug, Dox encapsulated Green-TiO_2 labeled as D_1, D_2, D_3, D_4 for the pH 3.0, 6.0, 8.0 and 10.0 respectively. The scheme of Drug Encapsulation over Green-TiO_2 is shown in fig. 6.

3.5 Study on Cytotoxicity

3.5.1 Preparation for testing cytotoxicity

The cytotoxicity of the test compound is analyzed in human cancer cell lines, HeLa cells using MTT colorimetric cell viability assay. The compound, 3-[4,5-dimethylthiazol-2-yl] 2,5-diphenyltetrazolium bromide (MTT) is a yellow coloured water soluble tetrazolium salt. During MTT assay mitochondrial enzyme in living cells, succinate-dehydrogenase, cleaves the tetrazolium ring present in the MTT compund converting the MTT to an insoluble purple formazan. Consequently the amount of formazan produced is directly proportional to the number of viable cells.

3.6 Cell culture

Human cervical cancer cell line (HeLa) obtained from National Centre for Cell Science (NCCS), Pune was grown in Eagles Minimum Essential Medium with 10% fetal bovine serum (FBS). The cells were maintained at $370°C$, 5% CO_2.

3.7 Cell treatment

The monolayer cells were detached with trypsin-ethylene diaminetetra acetic acid (EDTA) to make single cell suspensions and diluted with medium containing 5% FBS to get final density of $1x10^5$ cells/ml. One hundred micro litres per well of cell suspension were seeded into 96-well plates at plating density of 10,000 cells/well and incubated under the conditions of 37°C, 5% CO_2, 95% air and 100% relative humidity. After 24 h the cells were treated with serial concentrations of the test samples Bio-Extract, Green TiO_2 and DoX-encapsulated Green TiO_2. They were initially dispersed in phosphate buffered saline and an aliquot of the sample solution was diluted to twice the desired final maximum test concentration with serum free medium. Additional four serial dilutions were made to provide a total of five sample concentrations. Aliquots of 100 µl of these different sample dilutions were added to the appropriate wells containing 100 µl of medium with or without cells (blank), resulting in the required final sample concentrations. The medium containing without samples were served as positive control and triplicate was maintained for all concentrations. Following sample addition, the plates were incubated under the same conditions for an additional 48 h.

3.8 Cytotoxicity test

After the incubation period, 15µl of MTT (5mg/ml) in phosphate buffered saline (PBS) was added to each well and incubated at 37°C for 4h. Medium is aspirated and formazan crystals were dissolved in DMSO and absorbance is measured at 570nm using a micro plate reader. Cytotoxicity of any drug solution is usually measured in terms of cell viability. The percent cell inhibition or reduction in cell viability is determined using the following formula

$$\% \text{ Cell Inhibition} = \frac{100 - \text{treated}}{\text{Control}} \times 100$$

3.9 Experimental and characterization techniques

The Green-TiO_2 and the drug DoX encapsulated Green - TiO_2 were subjected to different experimental and characterization technique to investigate the morphological and structural properties.

3.9.1 UV- Absorption Spectroscopy

The principle of UV-Vis spectroscopy is based on the ability of molecule to absorb uv and visible light. The absorption of light corresponds to the excitation of outer electrons in the molecule. When a molecule absorbs energy and the outer electrons in the molecule excited from the Highest Occupied Molecular Orbital (HOMO) to Lowest Unoccupied Molecule Orbital (LUMO). The molecular orbital's with lowest energy are known the σ orbital's, at slightly higher energy are called π orbital's and still higher energy are known non- bonding orbital's (unshared pair electrons). The π* and σ* are called the highest energy state. [Pavia et al, 1997].

The absorption can be measured at a single wavelength or on spectral extended range. Ultraviolet and Visible spectroscopy are enough energetic to excite outer electrons to high energy level and it is very useful for quantity measurement. The Beer – Lambert Law is used to determine the concentration of analyze by measuring the absorbance at various wavelengths. Beer – Lambert Law is the relationship between absorbance and concentration.

It can be written as,

$$A = \varepsilon \, cl.$$

Where 'A' is the absorbance, 'ε' is the molar absorbtivity and expressed in units L mol^{-1} cm^{-1}, 'c' is the concentration of the sample (compound) and expressed as mol L^{-1} and 'l' is length of cell and expressed in units cm [Pavia et al, 1997]

3.9.2 UV -Vis Spectra

Absorption spectra were recorded by using UV-Vis spectrophotometer (Mode UV -2101 PC Shimadzu). The light generated from a Xenon flash lamp and is passed through the monochromator which splits the beam into different wavelengths out of the continuous spectrum. The intensity '10' measured by the fraction of beam redirected using beam splitter. The transmitted intensity 'I' of the light beam is measured at photo detector and the absorbance is calculated by the following formula.

$$A = log \ \frac{Io}{I}$$

The absorption is plotted as a function of the wavelength in an absorption spectrum. The molar absorptivity is calculated by using the Beer – Lambert law.

3.9.3 Fourier transformation IR Spectroscopy

Infrared spectra were performed with a Fourier transform infrared (FT-IR) spectrometer (Shimadzu, Model 8400S). The prepared samples were characterized by FTIR spectroscopy. The dried powder was properly mixed with KBr matrix. The translucent disks were prepared by pressing the ground material with the aid of 8-tonnes pressure bench press. The tablet was immediately analyzed with a spectrophotometer in the range of 4000-400 cm^{-1} with a resolution of $4cm^{-1}$. The IR radiation is passed through a sample. Some of the infrared radiation is absorbed by the sample and some of it is passed through (transmitted). The resulting spectrum represents the molecular absorption and transmission, gives information of type of bonding in the sample. This makes infrared spectroscopy useful for several types of analysis.

- FTIR can identify unknown materials
- FTIR can determine the quality or consistency of a sample
- FTIR can determine the amount of components in a mixture.

The original infrared instruments were of the dispersive type. These instruments separated the individual frequencies of energy emitted from the infrared source. This was accomplished by the use of a prism or grating. A grating is a more modern dispersive element which better separates the frequencies of infrared energy.

The detector measures the amount of energy at each frequency which has passed through the sample. This results in a spectrum which is a plot of intensity vs. frequency. Fourier Transform Infrared (FT-IR) spectrometry was developed in order to overcome the limitations encountered with dispersive instruments. The main difficulty was the slow scanning process. A method for measuring all of the infrared frequencies simultaneously, rather than individually, was needed. A solution was developed which employed a very simple optical device called an interferometer. The interferometer produces a unique type of signal which has all of the infrared frequencies "encoded" into it. The signal can be measured very quickly, usually on the order of one second. Thus the time element per sample is reduced to a matter of a few seconds rather than several minutes.

Infrared spectroscopy (IR) is mostly used by organic and inorganic chemists. In very simple way, it is the absorption measurement of IR frequencies of the sample positioned in the path of IR beam. Organic and Inorganic molecules absorbed IR radiations and converted it into vibration, stretching and bending molecular energy. Different functional groups and bonds absorbed infra red radiation at various wavelengths.

Electromagnetic radiations lower in energy than visible radiations are called infrared radiations. The electromagnetic spectrum of infrared region is divided into three parts, the near-, the mid-, and far- infra red region. The near – infrared region lies between $14000 – 4000 \text{ cm}^{-1}$, mid region between $4000 - 200 \text{ cm}^{-1}$ and far region $200 - 10 \text{ cm}^{-1}$. When the electromagnetic radiations of Infrared region are fall on the molecule, it absorbed the energy and the amount of absorbed energy is enough for the vibration motion of molecule. The energy which is not absorbed is transmitted through the sample. A graph plotted between absorbance and wave number is known as infrared spectrum.

A bond in an organic molecule may either stretch or bend with respect to other bonds. In stretching vibration, the inter – nuclear distances between two atoms increases or decreases but the atoms remain at the same bond axis.

3.9.4 X-ray Diffraction

The crystal structural investigations of the samples were performed on a Shimadzu model XRD 6000 X-ray diffractometer with Cu Kα line. X-ray diffraction (XRD) is a versatile, non-destructive technique used for qualitative and quantitative analysis of a crystalline materials. This experimental technique has been used to determine the overall structure of bulk solids, including lattice constants, identification of unknown materials, orientation of single crystals, orientation of polycrystalline, stress, texture, films thickness etc. in this study a power diffraction system with Cu-Kα X-Ray tube (λ=1.54056 A0) A was used. The X-Ray scans were performed between 2θ values of 30° and 80° with a typical step size of about 0.1° [39, 40].

3.9.4.1 Generation of X –ray

X-rays are short-wavelength, high energy electromagnetic radiation, having the properties of both waves and particles. They can be described in terms of both photon energy (E) or wavelength, λ (lambda – the distance between peaks) and frequency ν (nu – the number of peaks passing a point in a unit of time).

X-Rays are produced whenever high energy electrons strike with metal target, any x-ray tube must contain (a) a source of electron (b) a high accelerating voltage (c) a metal target. All x-ray tubes contain two electrodes, an anode (the metal target) usually maintained, at ground potential, and a cathode maintained at the negative potential, normally of order of 30KV to 50KV for the diffraction work. Interaction that occur between the beam (i.e. electron) and target will result in a loss of energy. A continuous spectrum is formed when the high energy electrons are slowed down rapidly by multiple collisions with the anode material, which give rise to white radiation, or so called Bremsstrahlung.

The continuous spectrum is formed due to rapid deceleration of the electrons hitting the target, as mentioned above, but not every electron decelerates in the same way, some stop in one impact and release all their energy at once, while other deflect this way and they encounter atoms of the target, successively losing fractions of their total kinetic energy until all is spent. Those electrons which are stopped in one impact produce photons of maximum energy (wavelength) equal to the energy loss.

3.9.4.2 Crystallite size measurement

Phase identification using x-ray diffraction depends on the positions of the peaks in a diffraction profile as well as the relative intensities of these peaks to some extent. Another aspect of the diffraction from material is the importance to consider how diffraction peaks are changed by the presence of various types of defects such as small number of dislocations in crystals with dimensions of millimeters. Small size of grain size can be considered as another kind of defect and can change diffraction peak widths. Very small crystals cause peak boarding. The crystallite size is easily calculated as a function of peak width (specified as the full- width at half maximum peak intensity (FWHM), peak position and wavelength.

3.9.4.3 Scherer's formula

Suppose that the crystal has a thickness d measured in a direction perpendicular to a particular set of Bragg planes.

Bragg angle as a variable and let θB be the angle which exactly satisfies Bragg's law for the particular values of λ and d involved, or

$$n\lambda = 2d \sin\theta$$

3.9.4.4 Determination of lattice parameters:

For the quartzite structure the inter planar distance of (hkl) plane is related to the lattice Parameters a and c via the Miller indices hkl.

3.9.5. Scanning electron microscopy (SEM) and Energy-dispersive X-ray spectroscopy (EDX)

3.9.5.1 Scanning Electron Microscope

The morphology and size distribution of the as-prepared samples were examined by using JEOL model JSM 6360 model Scanning Electron Microscope. The scanning electron microscope (SEM) is a type of electron microscope that helps in forming an image of the sample surface by scanning. The electrons in the beam interact with the atoms in the surface to generate signals that shed valuable light properties like composition, topography and electrical conductivity. The so called "signals" produced by an SEM include secondary and black- scattered electrons, characteristic x-rays, specimen current and light (due to cathode luminescence). All SEMs usually have the ability to detect secondary electrons but it's highly unlikely that a single SEM will have the ability to detect all the signals mentioned above. SEM helps in obtaining high resolution images of specimens ranging in size from those visible to the naked eye to those which are just a few nanometers in size.

In most of the applications, the data collected is over a pre selected area of the sample surface and following this, a 2D image is generated that shows the various spatial variations. Conventional SEMs with a magnification range of 20X-30000X with a spatial resolution of 50-100 nm can scan areas which vary from 1cm to 5 μm in width. SEMs also have the ability to analyze particular points as can be seen during EDX operations which help in determining the chemical composition of the sample concerned. Secondary electrons and back scattered electrons are most commonly used for the purpose of imaging samples, secondary electrons depict morphology and topography of the samples while back scattered electrons depict contrasts in composition in multiphase samples. X-Rays are produced when incident electrons collide in elastically with the electrons of the atoms in the sample. As the excited electrons get back to their previous positions, they emit x-rays which is the characteristic property of a material. SEM analysis is said to be a non destructive analysis as the bombardment of electrons do not cause any damage to the samples.

Essential components of all SEMs include the following:

- Electron Source ("Gun")
- Electron Lenses
- Sample Stage
- Detectors for all signals of interest
- Display / Data output devices
- Infrastructure Requirements:
- Power Supply
- Vacuum System
- Cooling system
- Vibration-free floor
- Room free of ambient magnetic and electric fields

Sample preparation is not really a problem in case of SEM analysis as the only requirement for a sample to undergo SEM analysis is that it should be conductive. It also allows a large amount of the sample to be focused at once as it has a large depth of field in analyzing the spatial features closely. A combination of all these features has made the SEM one of the most popular instruments in the world on materials science.

3.9.5.2 Energy Dispersive X-Ray Spectroscopy

Energy dispersive X-Ray analysis, also known as EDS, EDX or EDAX, is a technique used to identify the elemental composition of a sample. During EDS, a sample is exposed to an electron beam inside a scanning electron microscope (SEM). These electrons collide with the electrons within the sample, causing some of them to be knocked out of their orbits. The vacated positions are filled by higher energy electrons which emit X-Rays in the process. By analyzing the emitted X-Rays, the elemental composition of the sample can be determined. EDS is a very handy tool for performing the constitutional analysis of any kind of material.

3.9.6. High Resolution Imaging (HRTEM)

The particle size, morphology, lattice fringe and selected area Electron Diffraction pattern of the samples were characterized using a JOEL 2010, Tecnai F-20 Transmission Electron Microscope. This work uses HRTEM in the conventional sense to generate the images but employs a novel technique in the image interpretation. The HRTEM images were used to generate strain maps over the quantum well regions.

CHAPTER 4

RESULTS AND DISCUSSIONS

4.1 Characterization of Artemisia Pallens plant extract.

4.1.1 GC-MS chromatogram of Artemisia pallens

The GC-MS chromatogram of the Artemisia Pallens water extracts is represented in Fig.7. It showed 7 prominent peaks with very narrow retention time. The fragmentation patterns for some of the peaks were comparable with the standard compounds. Data shown in Table 1.1 revealed that the derivative of the compound 5-hepten-3-one was predominantly present in water based extract with the retention time of 17.12 min. This compound shows a molecular ion peak at 236 and a base peak at 111, (WILEY8.LIE CAS: 20482-11-5). The second largest compound extracted out with the retention time of 6.64 min was found to be 5, 5-Dimethyl-2(5H)-Furanone. This derivative shows a molecular ion peak at 112 and a base peak at 97.05, (WILEY8. LIE CAS: 20019-64-1). The third major derivative extracted out with retention time at 2.41 min was found to be 2-pentanol. This compound has a molecular ion peak at 73 and a base peak at 45.0, (WILEY8.LIE CAS: 6032-29- 7). It is expected that these three major compounds present in the water-based extract from the plant material are responsible for the hydrolysis and condensation reactions of the precursors of TiO_2.

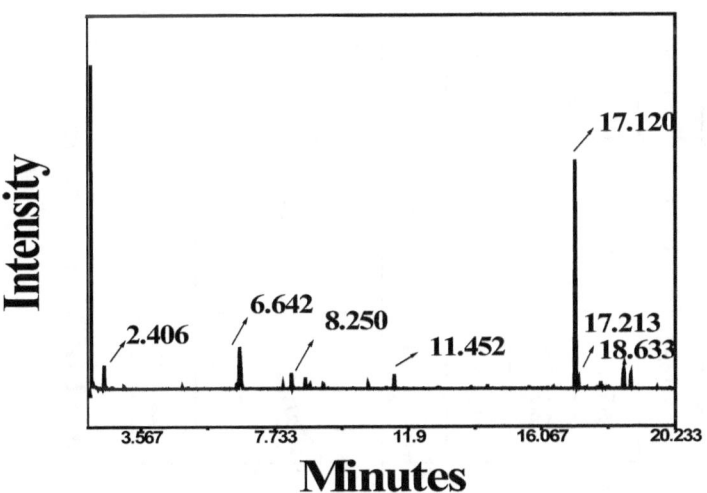

Fig.7 GCMS spectrum of Artemisia pallens extract

Peak	R.Time	Area	Area%	Height	Height%	A/H	Name
1	2.406	58191	4.59	34623	6.03	1.68	2-PENTANOL
2	6.644	216359	17.07	65116	11.34	3.32	2(5H)-FURANONE
3	8.250	42213	3.33	23240	4.05	1.82	2(3H)-FURANONE
4	11.452	31477	2.48	21733	3.79	1.45	ETHANONE
5	17.120	771165	60.84	360771	62.84	2.14	5-HEPTEN-3-ONE
6	18.633	79423	6.27	30677	5.34	2.59	2-(1-HYDROXY ETHYL)-5-METHYL-5-VINYL-TETRAHYDROFURAN
7	18.855	35064	2.77	21124	3.68	1.68	4-HEPTEN-3-ONE

Table.1 GCMS peak report

4.1.2 FTIR Spectrum of Artemisia Pallens plant extracts

The FTIR spectrum of Artemisia Pallens plant extract is in Fig.8. The strong absorption band appeared at $3361.93cm^{-1}$ arise due to polymeric structure of intermolecular OH stretching vibrations due to free hydroxyl present in plant extract. This is further confirmed by GCMS data given in Table:1 indicating the presence of 2-Pentanol with retention time2.408 min and molecular ion peak at 73 and base peak at 45. The band at $2970.38cm^{-1}$ corresponds to asymmetric C-H stretching. A small sharp peak was observed at $1641.42cm^{-1}$ was observed and can be attributed to the presence of aromatic ring. A significant small ketonic derivative peak observed at 1627.92 cm^{-1}. This peak at $1627.92cm^{-1}$ present in *Artemisia pallens* plant extract indicating the presence of ketonic derivatives can be confirmed by GCMS data given in Table:1 which shows the presence of the 5-hepten-3-one with retention time 17.12 min and molecular ion peak at 236 and base peak at 111. Other ketonic derivatives given in GCMS Data are 5,5-Dimethyl-2(5H)-Furanone with retention time 6.64 and molecular ion peak at 112 and base peak at 43. Absorption peak at 2310.72 cm^{-1} is due to atmospheric carbondioxide impurity.

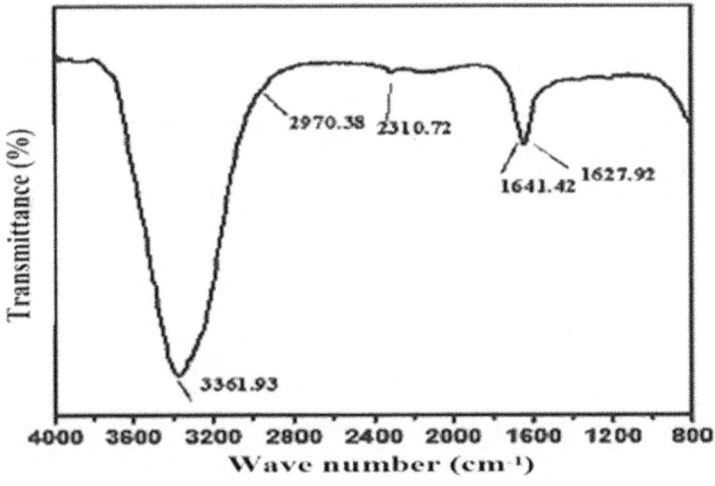

Fig.8 FTIR spectrum of Artemisia pallens plant extract

4.2 Green TiO$_2$ – Characterization

4.2.1 U V

Figure 9(a) shows the DRS spectrum of Green TiO$_2$. It shows that the Green-TiO$_2$ absorbs only in the uv range less than 410nm. The excited photon energy of Green-TiO2 having longitude close to 410nm, having band gap of 3.2 ev. The literature reports 3.23 electron volts for anatase phase [M. Litter 1999, Sergio Valencia *et al.,* (2013)]. The Green-TiO$_2$ shows absorption band centered at 310-320nm, which is attributed to the presence of isolated poly titanate framework (Ti-O-Ti)$_n$ [S. Klein *et al.,* (1996); G.Petrini, *et al.,* (1991); Mohamed S. Hamdy (2014)].

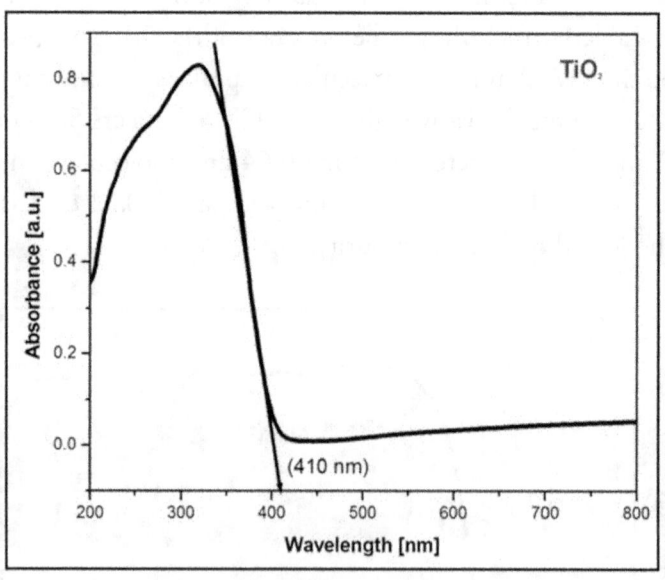

Fig.9 (a) UV- Vis Diffuse Reflectance spectra of Green TiO$_2$ Nanoparticle

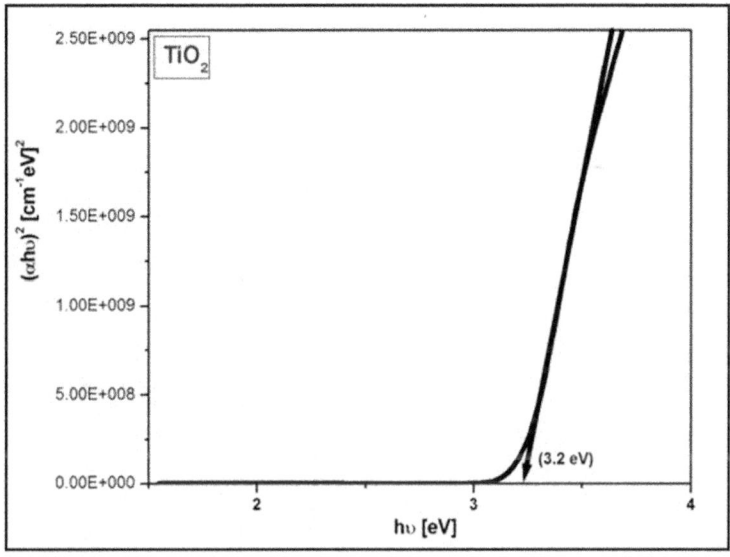

Fig.9 (b) Band gap of Green TiO$_2$ Powder sample

4.2.2 FTIR

Figure 10 shows FTIR spectra of TiO$_2$ nano-particles. The spectrum shows a band at 435 cm^{-1} corresponding to metal–oxygen (Ti–O). The hydroxyl group band found in IR spectrum of *Artemisia pallens* plant extract is not observed in IR spectrum of TiO$_2$ nano-particles. This clearly indicates that after calcinations, there are no traces of hydroxyl group and synthesized TiO$_2$ nano-particles is pure. The band at 1618cm^{-1} is attributed to presence plane bending vibrations of O-H and CO$_2$ molecules. The absorption band at 1438 cm^{-1} might be expected to be C-O-H bending band, usually appears near 1440-1395cm^{-1} with moderate intensity and occurs in the same region as the CH$_2$ scissoring vibration of the CH$_2$ group adjacent to the carbonyl.

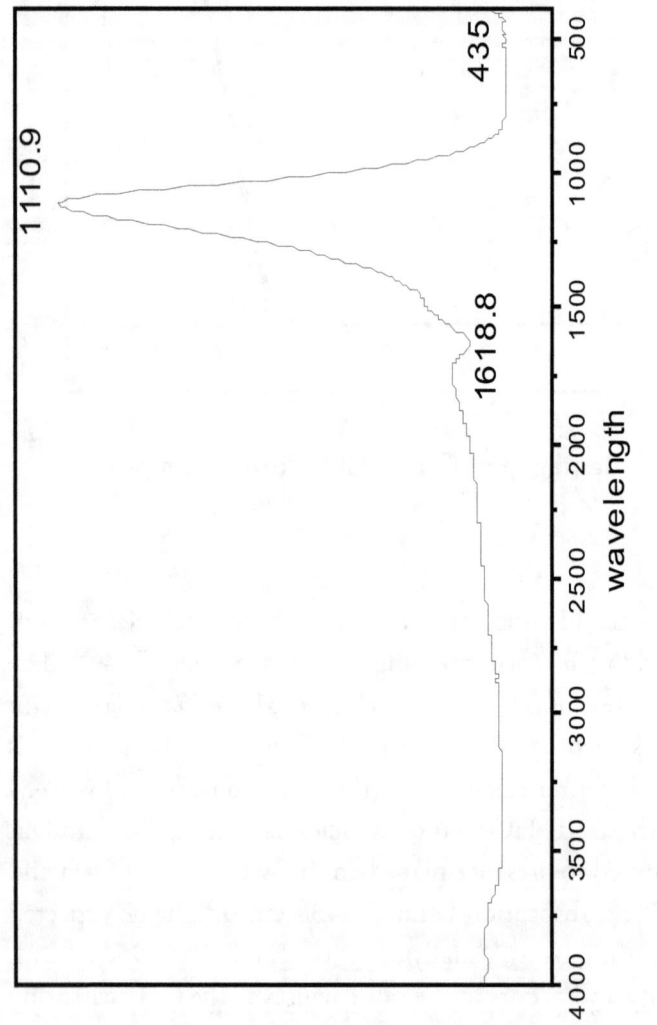

Fig.10 FTIR Spectrum of Green TiO₂ Nano Particles

4.2.3 XRD

Figure 11 shows XRD pattern of the TiO_2 nano-particles. There are two prominent peaks observed at 2θ = 25.65°, 48.37° and corresponds to (101), (200) reflection. The other diffraction peaks observed at 2θ=38.2°, 54.0°, 55.3°, 63.3°, 70.7° and 75.0°, corresponds to (004), (105), (211), (204) (220), (215) planes are also observed. The crystallite size was calculated using Debye-Scherer equation and found to be 9-16 nm. The spherical shape of TiO_2 nano-particles is observed from the diffraction pattern. The diffraction patterns matches with the standard JCPDS card no 89-4921.

The lattice constants, a and c of as-synthesized TiO_2 nanoparticles were calculated using Bragg's law and found to be a=4.0055 Å, c=6.9378 Å.

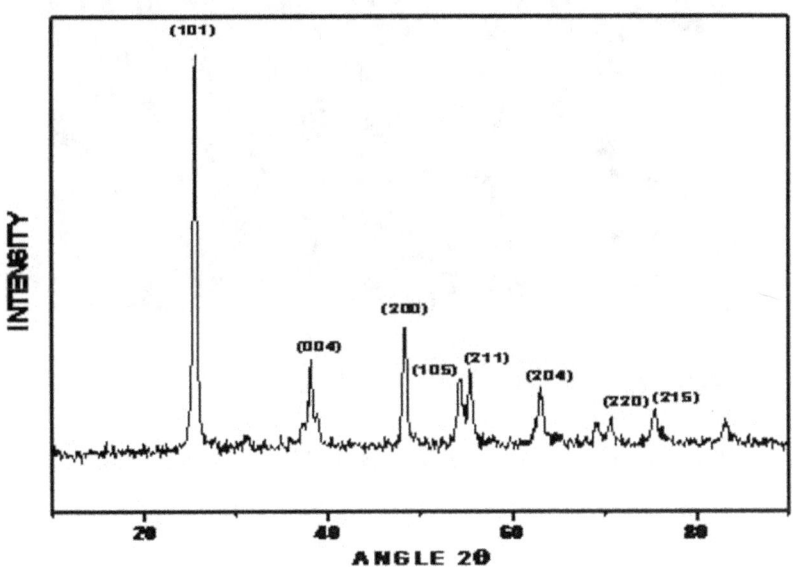

Fig.11 XRD Spectrum of Green TiO$_2$ Nano Particles

4.2.4: EDX

The EDS of as- synthesized TiO_2 is shown in Fig 12. It is seen from the spectrum, the as-synthesized using green solvent shows only titanium and oxygen elements, suggesting 100% purity of the as-synthesizes TiO_2. The EDS spectrum indicates 48.2% of titanium and 52.8% of oxygen contribute to 100% of the total weight. This confirms the purity of TiO_2 nano-particles by sol-gel route using green solvent is good.

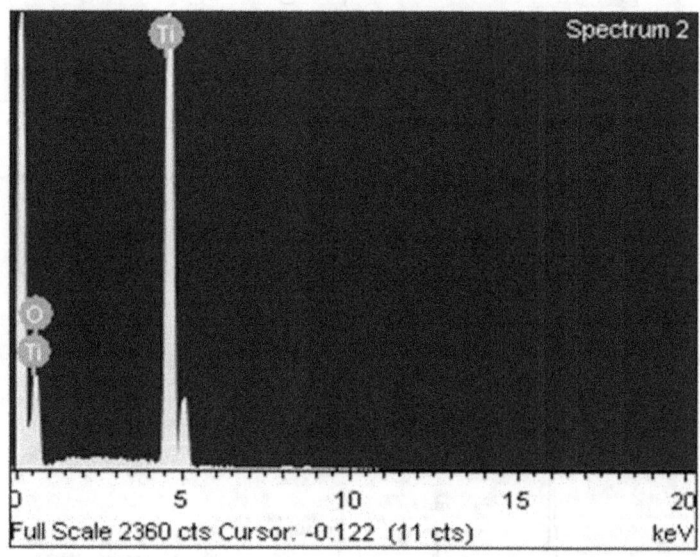

Fig.12 EDX Spectrum of Green TiO_2 Nano Particles

S.No	Compound	Percentage %
1	Titanium	48.2
2	Oxygen	52.8

Table 2: EDX peak report of Green TiO_2

4.2.5: SEM

The SEM image of TiO$_2$ nano powders is shown in Fig 13. The green synthesized TiO$_2$ nano-particle by sol-gel method shows the tetragonal shape of various sizes. The TiO$_2$ nano-particles have aggregated to form the nano clusters. The average crystalline size of TiO$_2$ is not clearly seen in image due to agglomeration of the nano particles. The particle morphology was obtained by SEM image

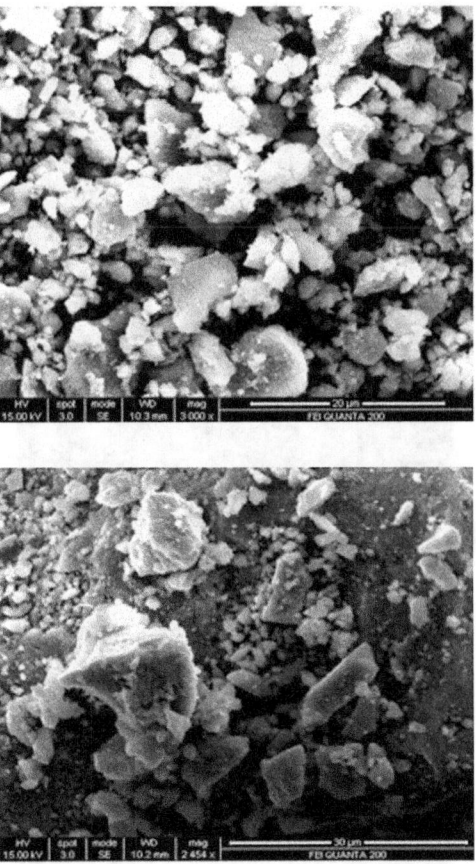

Fig.13 SEM images of Green TiO$_2$ Nano Powder

4.2.6 TEM

TEM Image of TiO_2 nano-powder is presented in Fig 15(a). The particle size, crystallinity and the morphology can be obtained from TEM images. It is revealed from the images the mean particle range from 9-16nm shown in Fig 15(b) with hexagonal in shape. The Selective Area Diffraction Pattern SAED shown in Fig 14 was in good agreement with the XRD observations. The characteristic diffraction rings corresponding to anatase phase were seen in SAED pattern.

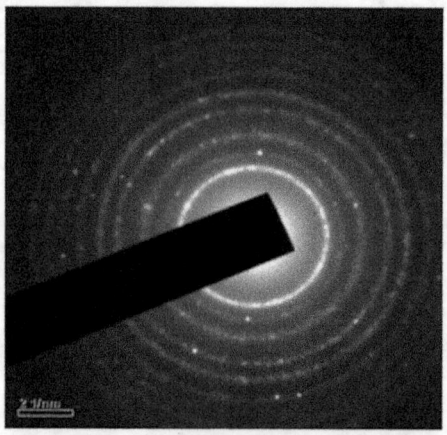

Fig. 14 SAED Pattern of Green TiO_2 nano powder

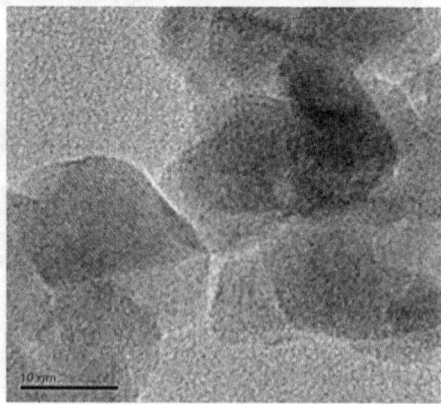

Fig.15 (a) TEM Image of Green TiO_2 nano powder

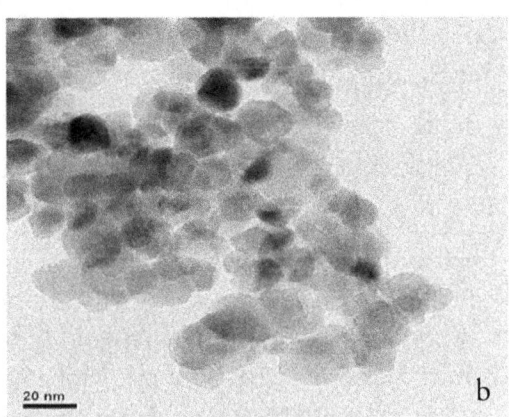

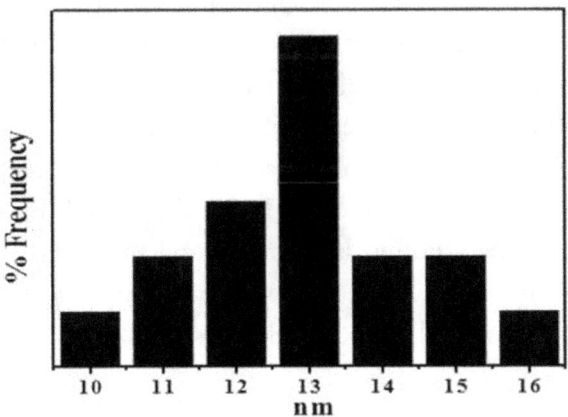

**Fig.15 (b) Tem Image of Green TiO$_2$ nano powder
and average particle size**

4.3 Loading of DoX on Green - TiO$_2$

4.3.1 Different pH at Different Equilibration time:

Figure 16 shows the UV-Vis absorbance spectra of the supernatant solution of the mixture of Green TiO$_2$ and DoX, drug at different pH values at different time intervals. Fig 16 a,b,c,d shows the effect of pH 3,6,8 & 10 at different equilibration time.

Comparing the fig a and d, the maximum absorbance of drug at 483 nm shows lesser intensity. It suggests that the stability of the drug at Ph 3.0 and 10.0 is doubtful. It reveals from Fig.16 b and Fig.16 c the maximum intensity was observed suggesting better stability of the DoX drug. Further analysis of the Fig. 16 b and Fig.16 c, the intensity of the supernatant obtained after the different time intervals, shows gradual decrease in the absorbance at 483nm. [Mohammed Ghanbari *et al.,* (2016)] It seems that at 18 hours of equilibration time shows no traces of DoX in the supernatant suggesting, complete transfer of DoX over Green TiO$_2$. It may be concluded that, the drug DoX loading over Green- TiO$_2$ at pH 6.0 and 8.0 seems to be more effective at 18 hours of equilibration time compared to pH 3.0 and 10.0.

In Fig.16 the pH was obtained naturally 6.0 by mixing of DoX with distilled water, where as in 16.c the DoX solution pH was regulated to 8.0 using phosphate buffer. It is understood from Fig16.b was more effective in natural pH, hence further cyto-toxicity analysis was carried out at pH 6.0 and equilibrated at 18 hours.

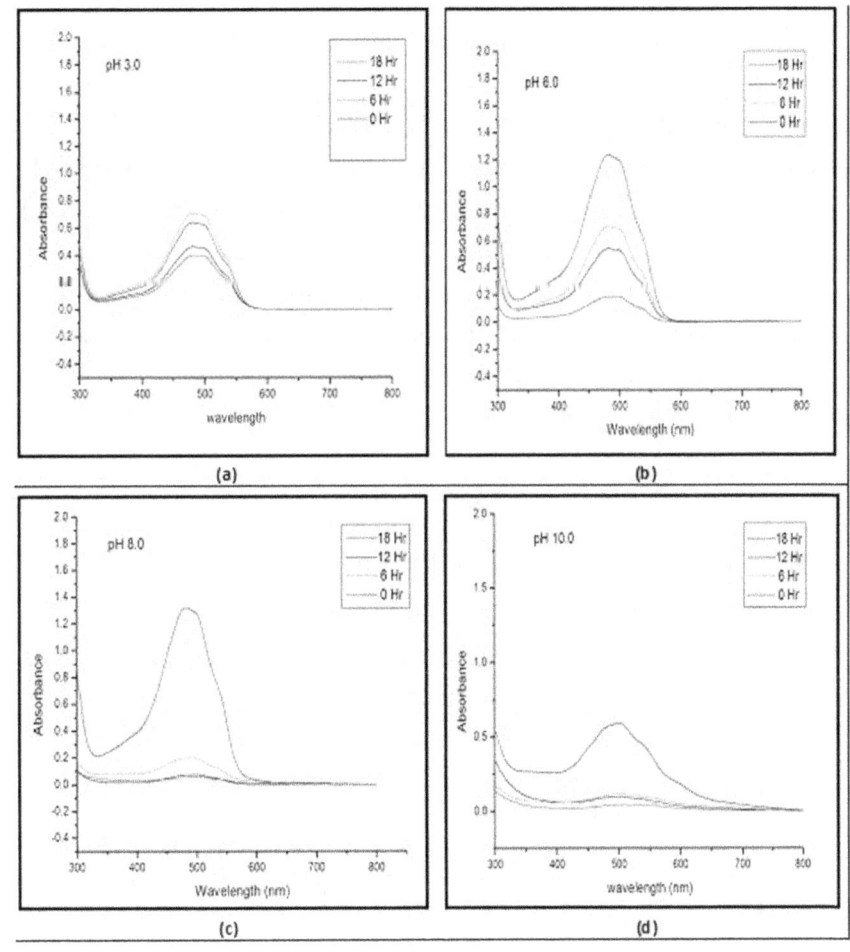

Fig.16 Absorbance peak of Doxorubicin Doped TiO₂ of Ph 3.0, 6.0, 8.0 and 10.0

4.4 TiO$_2$-DoX- Characterization

4.4.1 XRD

The XRD pattern of TiO$_2$ and DoX loaded on Green-TiO$_2$ (TiO$_2$-Dox) are shown in Fig. 17. The XRD pattern indicates good crystalline in nature. The diffraction peaks can be indexed as (101), (200) & (004) suggesting tetragonal anatase TiO$_2$ (JCPDS card 89-4921). While loading with DoX on TiO$_2$ there is a small shift was observed in all the diffraction peaks. This confirms the incorporation of DoX on TiO$_2$ lattice. Further the formation and the crystallization of TiO$_2$-Dox were confirmed through the lattice parameter and crystallite size values. The average crystallite size was calculated by using Debye Scherrer equation and found to be 10 and 13 nm for Green TiO$_2$ and TiO$_2$-DoX, respectively.

$$Dp = 0.94\lambda / \beta \cos\theta$$

Where, λ is the wavelength of the radiation (1.5406 Å), β is the full width half maximum (FWHM) and θ is the angle of diffraction. The increase in the value of crystallite size might be due to the loading effect of DoX on TiO$_2$. Lattice constants for Green TiO$_2$ and TiO$_2$-DoX are shown in Table. A new broad peak was observed at an angle 45.4° marked as arrow, reveals the crystallization of drug DoX over Green TiO$_2$.

Compound	Lattice Parameters		Cell Volume Å	Crystallite size (nm)
	A	C		
Green TiO$_2$	3.777	9.501	117.38	10
Green TiO$_2$-DoX	3.52	9.46	101.51	13

Table 3: Lattice parameter, Cell Volume and Crystallite size of Green TiO$_2$ and Green TiO$_2$-DoX

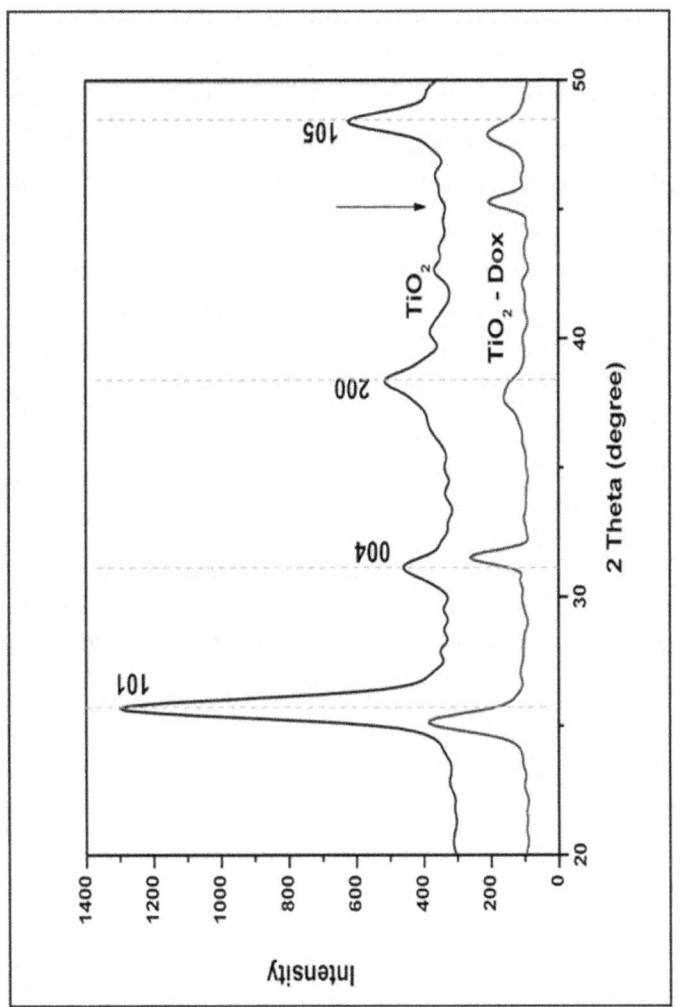

Fig.17 XRD pattern of Green-TiO$_2$ and Dox-TiO$_2$

4.4.2 FT-IR Analyses of Green TiO_2- DoX

The bonding formation between TiO_2 and DoX were studied through FTIR analysis and respective spectra of TiO_2, DoX and TiO_2 – DoX were shown in Fig 18. From Fig 18 (TiO_2), small peak was observed in the range of 480 cm^{-1} (centered at the far IR Region) is likely due to the vibration frequency of the Ti–O bonds in the TiO_2 lattice. Also, sharp peak was observed at 1618 cm^{-1} is assigned to the intercalated Ti-O-Ti bending vibration. In pure doxorubicin (DOX), characteristic peak was observed at 3062, 1336 and 906 cm^{-1}. This may be due to the –O-H / -N-H stretching, C=O stretching and C-Cl bending vibration (DoX in HCl), respectively. In TiO_2 – DOX, the FTIR spectrum shows some specific characteristic bands was observed at 3853 (Asymmetric amide -N-H Stretching), 3773 (Symmetric -O-H Stretching) and 1515 cm^{-1} (-N-O stretching vibration, strong band). The FTIR spectra of pure TiO_2 and DoX were compared with TiO_2-DoX in order to confirm their binding modes. The peaks observed from TiO_2 – DoX are not appeared in pure TiO_2 and DoX, which shows that the distortion in the pure structures. The observed frequencies are clearly indicates that the bond formation / loading of TiO_2 via the oxygen (from –C=O, -OH) and nitrogen (-NH). [Wenzhi Ren *et al.*, 2013; Mohammed Ghanbari *et al.*, 2016]

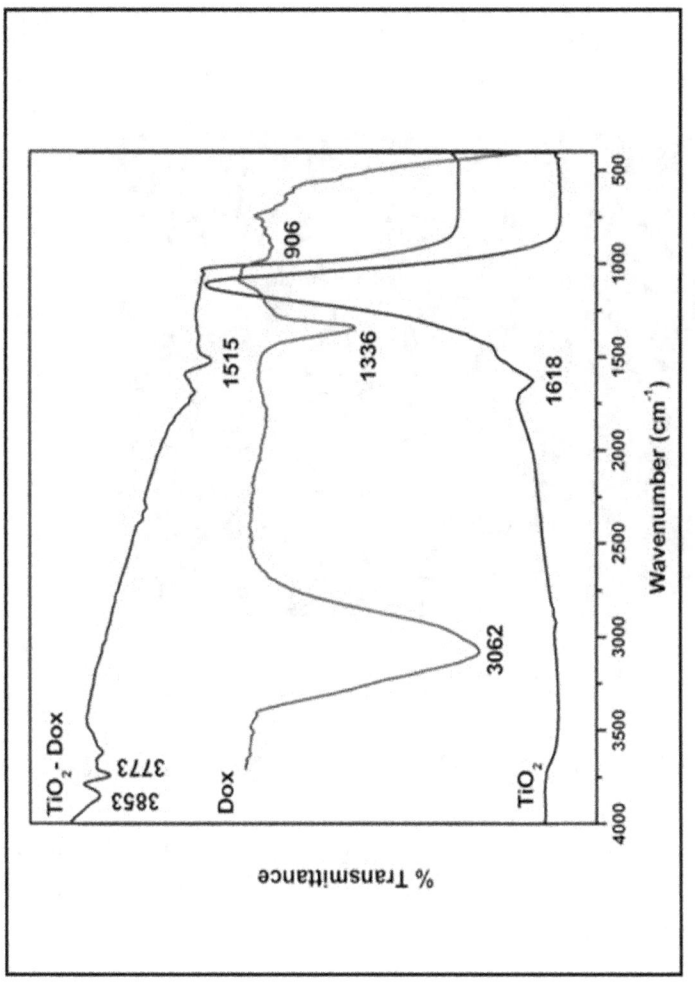

Fig. 18 FTIR spectra of Green-TiO$_2$, DOX and TiO$_2$-DOX

4.4.3: Green TiO₂-Dox EDX

The EDX spectrum results are shown in Fig.19 this spectrum shows elemental compositional peak of Titanium, oxygen, carbon and oxygen. This carbon and oxygen peak found in EDX of TiO_2-Dox is absent in EDAX spectrum of TIO_2 which indicates doping of doxorubicin drug to TiO_2 and presence of carbonyl groups in TiO_2–DoX. The composition of DoX-TiO_2 composition is shown in the following table.

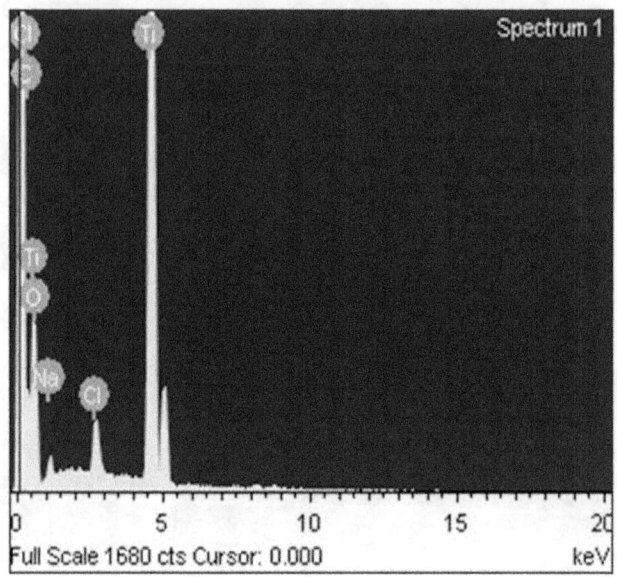

Fig.19 EDX Spectrum of Green TiO₂-DoX Nano particle

All the above observations conforms the doxorubicin drug loading into TiO_2 Nano particles. This emphasis that the solvent employed has influence in the synthesised nanocarrier.

4.4 Green TiO$_2$-Dox SEM

The SEM images of TiO$_2$-Dox shows even morphology when compared with the TiO$_2$ nano-powders. The doping of the docxorubicin drug has yielded a uniform adsorption of drug on TiO$_2$ and prevents the formation nano-clusters. This confirms the doxorubicin drug loaded into the TiO$_2$ nano-particles

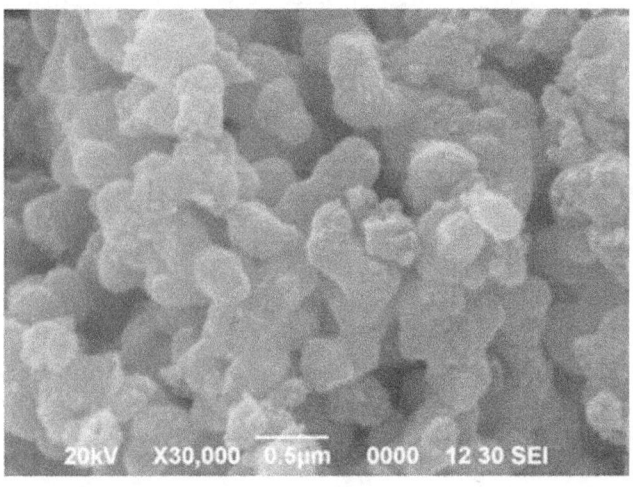

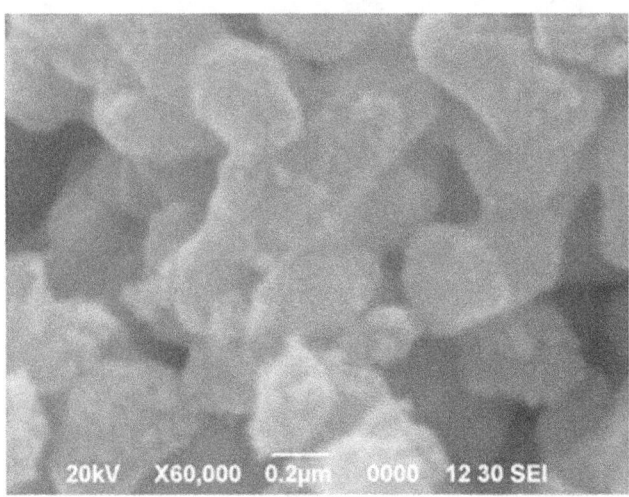

Fig.20 SEM Image of Green TiO$_2$-DoX nano particle

4.5 CELL-VIABILITY ANALYSIS

4.5.1 Effect of Green Solvent On Cell Viability

The effect of the concentration of Green Solvent used for the synthesis of TiO_2 nano carrier was examined to determine the cyto-toxicity on HeLA cells where shown in Fig.21. The figure represents the MTT assay in which MTT (3-[4,5-dimethylthiazol-2-yl]-2, 5-dophenyltetrazolium bromide) which is a water- soluble tetrazolium salt, and the assay is based on the principle that mitochondrial dehydrogenase of intact cells converts the soluble yellow MTT tetrazolium salt into an insoluble purple formazan through the cleavage of the tetrazoilum ring; the formazon product is impermeable to cell membranes with loss of integrity and therefore only accumulates in healthy cells (Shafiu Abdullahi Kamba *et al.,* 2013).

The figure reveals good cyto compatibility of the green solvent showed no toxicity to HeLa cells upto the concentration of 100 μl/ml and the cell viability was found to be around 98%.

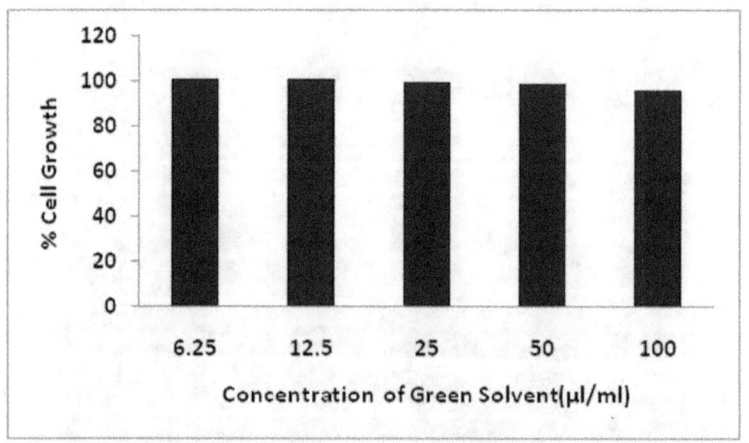

Fig.21 Cytotoxicity of Green solvent on HeLa cervical cancer cells line

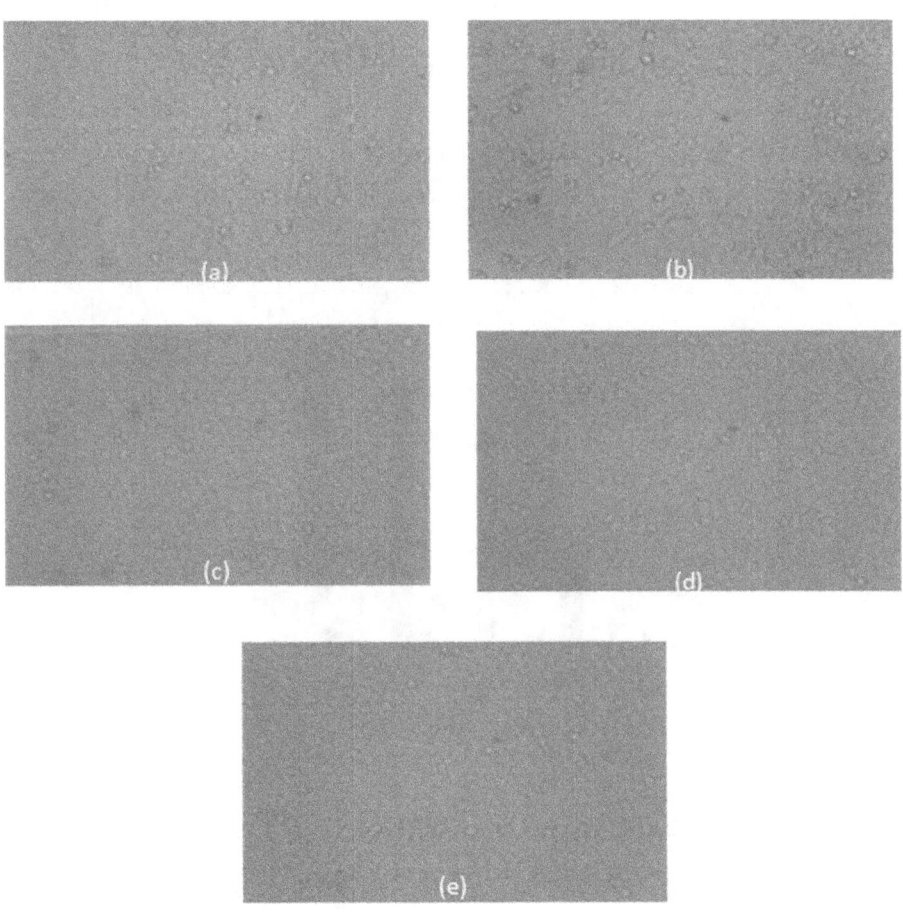

Fig.22 Images showing the effect of Green Solvent On Cell Viability(a)6.25, (b)12.5, (c)25, (d)50, (e)100 µl/ml

4.5.2 Effect of DoX on cell inhibition:

The cytotoxicity study of free DoX on HeLa cell was evaluated using an MTT assay. The cells were treated with different concentration of free DoX 0.005μg/ml, 0.05 μg/ml, 0.5 μg/ml, 5 μg/ml, 10 μg/ml and incubated for a period of 48 hours and shown in Fig. 23. It is observed from the figure that the cell inhibition depends on the concentration of DoX, the rate of inhibition increased with increase in the concentration of DoX under study. The IC 50 of free DoX against HeLa was found to be 0.28.

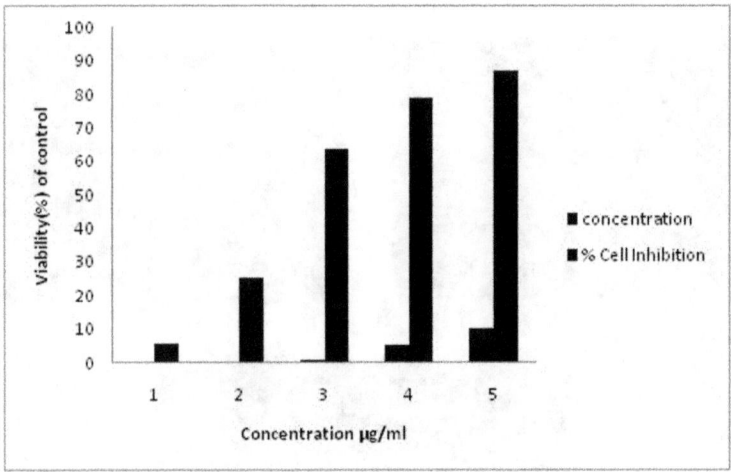

Fig.23 *In-vitro* cytotoxicity study of HeLa cervical cancer cells on exposure to free DoX

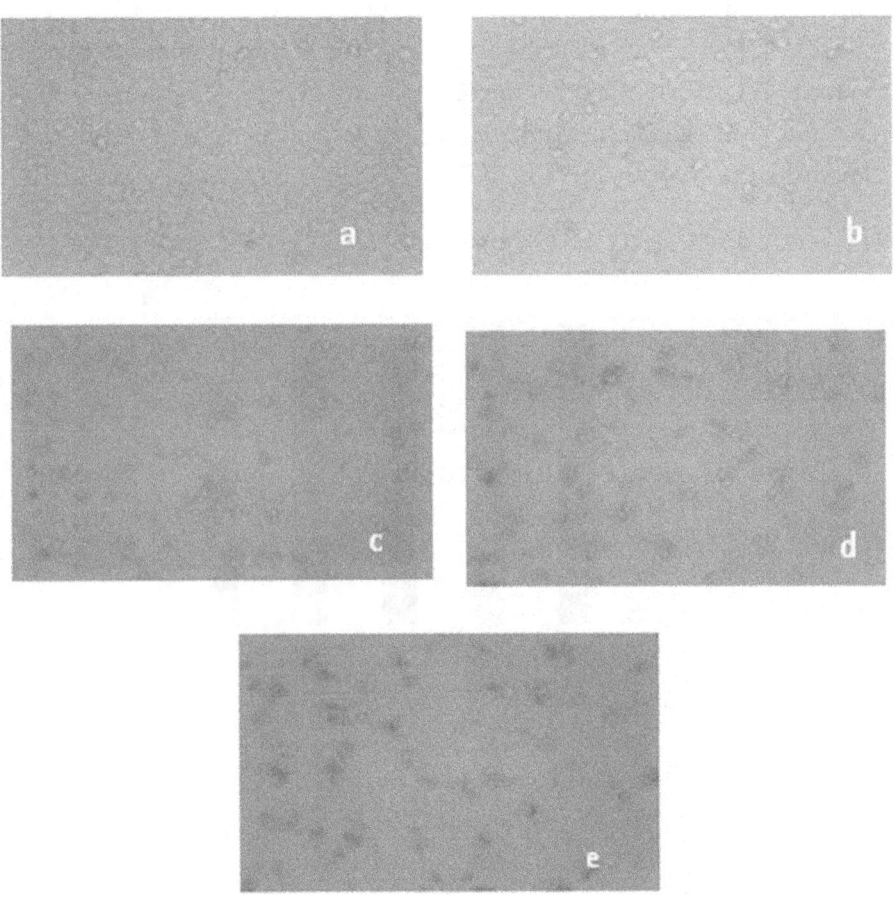

Fig.24 Effect of DoX on Cell inhibition (a) 0.005, (b) 0.05, (c) 0.5, (d) 5, (e) 50 μg/ml.

4.5.3 Effect of Green Synthesized TiO$_2$ on Cell Viability

The effect of different concentration of Green TiO$_2$ on HeLa cells incubated at 48hours is shown in Fig.25. The cell viability on the different concentration of Green TiO$_2$ was found to be 99.12, 99.41, 94.29, 87.93, and 81.06 % for 0.05. 0.5, 5, 50 and 100 µg/ml respectively. This result reveals a good cyto compatibility of green TiO$_2$ suggesting it has a potential Biomedical applications, especially as a carrier in the drug delivery system.

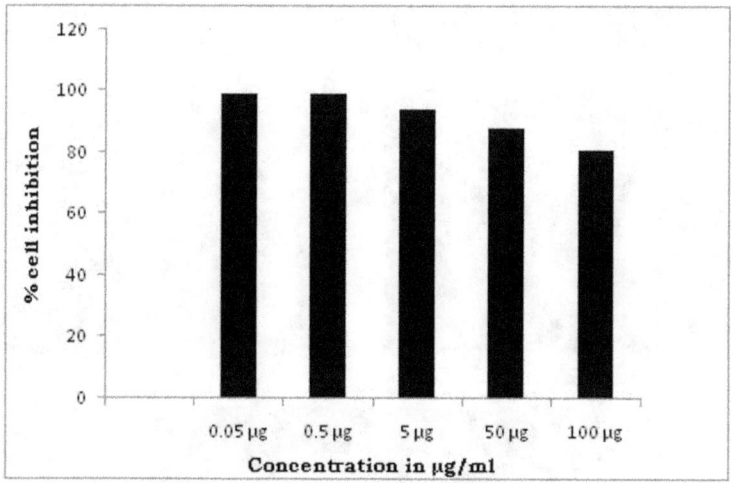

Fig.25 Cytotoxicity of Green TiO$_2$ on HeLa cervical cancer cell

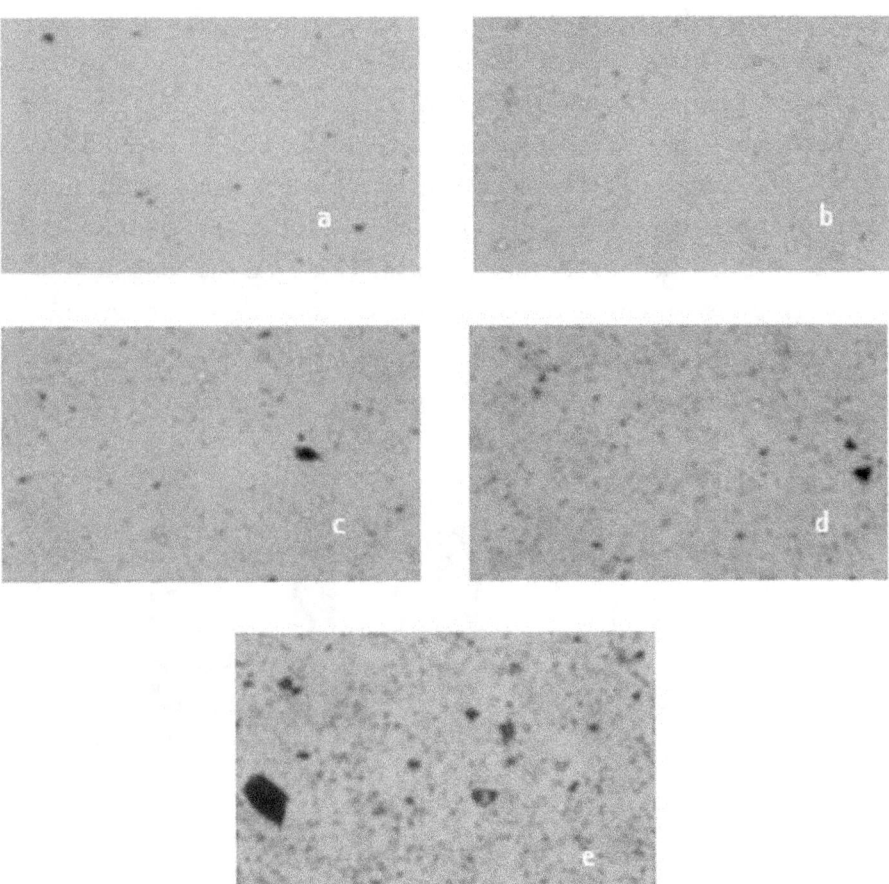

Fig.26 Cytotoxicity of Green-TiO$_2$ on HeLa(a) 12.5, (b) 25, (c) 50, (d) 100, (e) 200 μg/ml.

4.5.4 *Invitro* toxicity of Green TiO$_2$-DoX

The effect of the concentration of DoX loaded Green TiO$_2$ on the HeLa cell inhibition was shown in Fig.27. The percent cell inhibition was found to be 1.24, 7.16, 22.00, 34.28 for 0.5, 5, 50, 100 µg/ml respectively. The cellular uptake of free DoX occurs through a passive diffusion mechanism whereby it may be trapped at the P-gp junction and thereby affect the normal cells while in the case of Green TiO$_2$-DoX, the drug has to be released in a time dependent manner from TiO$_2$ nano particles before exerts its effects on the cells, therefore as the time increases the rate of drug release increases and the concentration also increases, inhibiting the cell growth in a time dependent manner.

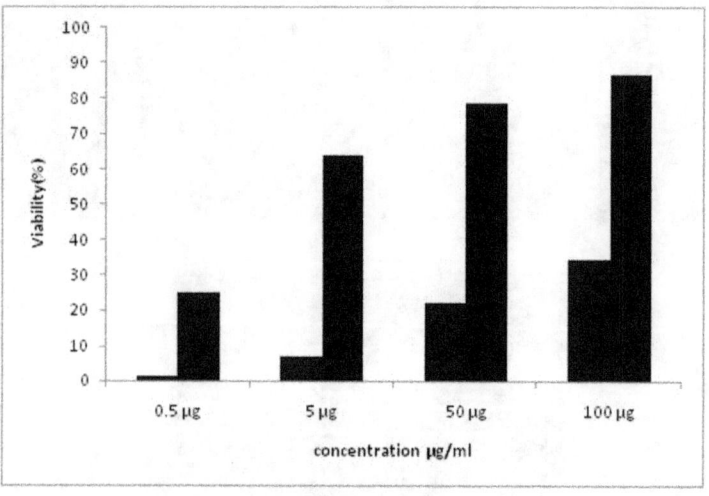

Fig.27 *Invitro* cyto toxicity study of HeLa cells after 48 hours of exposure to free DoX and Green TiO$_2$-DoX

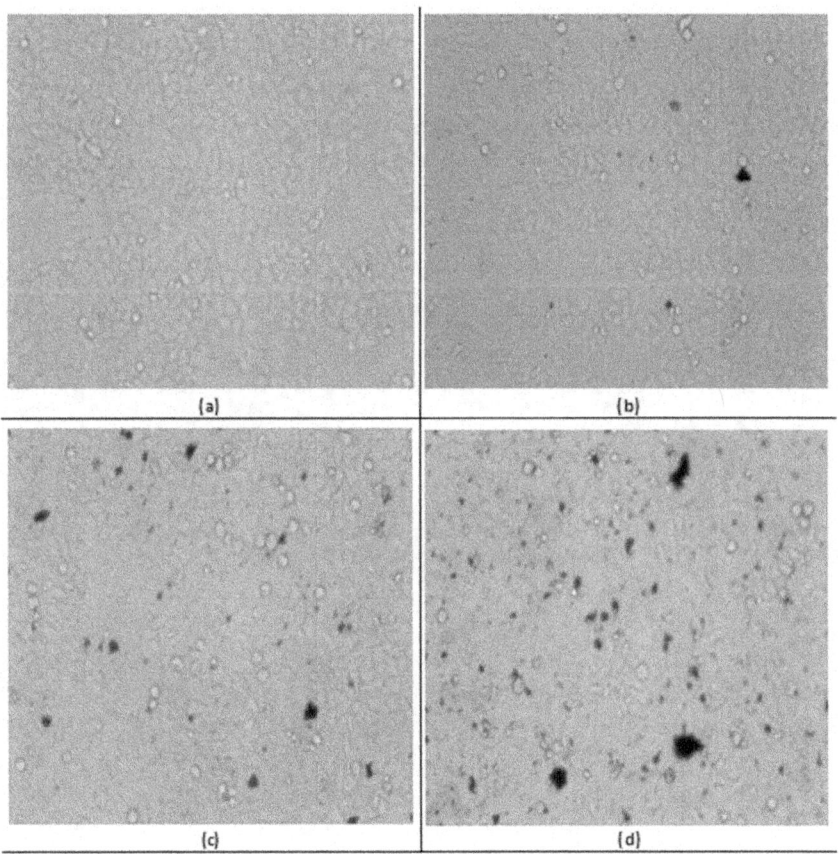

Fig.28 Showing *Invitro* toxicity studies of HeLa cells (a) 0.05,
(b) 5, (c) 50, (d) 100 µg/ml.

The cellular uptake of Green TiO_2-DoX nanocrystals was through non-specific endocytosis which may lead to reduced effect of cytosolic free DoX for the P-gp pumping action, this mechanism of Green TiO_2-DoX nanocrystal delivery to tumours may circumvent the effect of multidrug resistant proteins which are always present in the cancer cells [Gillies, E.R et al., 2005, Chittasupho, C et al., 2009]. P-glycoprotien has the capacity of recognizing drug and expelling them from the cancer cells only when such drugs are in the plasma membrane, and not when the drug is located in the cytoplasm of the lysosomes after endocytosis [Larsen A.K et al., 2000].

CHAPTER 5

* ━━━ ◄◎ ◎► ━━━ *

SUMMAARY AND CONCLUSION

Recently, considerable effort has been devoted to synthesize inorganic nanoparticles due to their unique physical properties compared to bulk materials. The unique properties of the nano materials make them very attractive in various applications including catalysis, high efficiency solar cells, coatings, cosmetics, sensors and drug delivery system

Among the nanoparticles reported in the literature, TiO_2 nano materials have received a great deal of attention due to their high activity, strong oxidation capability, and chemical stability. Different techniques have been practised for the sysnthesis of TiO_2-based nanostructures, such as anodization, template techniques, hydrothermal processes and soft chemical processes. However, each of these methods has its own limitations. For instance, the templating technique requires high calcinations temperature to remove the template, resulting in a collapse of the tubular structure of the synthesized materials. Anodizing produce nanotubes with relatively large diameters. The multi-step hydrothermal process requires a large amount of inorganic solvents, which are not eco-friendly. In this regard, the sol-gel technique using a green solvent considered to be an attractive alternate to synthesize TiO_2-based nano structured materials with desired characteristics.

5.1 Green synthesis

Developing reliable biosynthetic, an environment friendly approach has added much importance because of its ecofriendly products, biocompatibility and economic viability in the long run and also to avoid adverse effects during their application especially in medical field. The microbial enzyme or the plant phytochemicals with antioxidant or reducing properties are usually responsible for the preparation of metal and metal oxide nanoparticles. Recently nanoparticles synthesis were achieved with bacteria, fungi, use of plant extract such as neem, camellia sinensis, coriandrum, nelumbo lucifera, ocimum sanctum and several others which is compatible with the green chemistry principles. Among the various biosynthetic approaches, the use of plant extracts has advantage such as easily available, safe to handle and possess a broad viability of metabolites. The main phytochemicals responsible for the synthesis of nanoparticles are terpenoids, flavones, ketones, aldehydes amides etc. In continuation of the efforts for synthesizing titanium dioxide nanoparticle, here we reported a facile, green and one pot synthesis using the leaf extract of *Artemesia pallens* labeled Bio-Extract. *Artemesia pallens* has chosen because of its functional anti-inflammatory, antioxidant activities and synthesized TiO_2 labelled as Green-TiO_2.

5.2 Drug loading

We have loaded successfully the available anti cancer drug Doxorubicin (DoX) over the Green-TiO_2 nanoparticles at four different pH and optimized at its natural pH (6.0) of the drug. At this optimized condition, the texture of the product is found to be non-hygroscopic.

5.3 Characterization

In order to understand the composition of the phytochemicals, the *Artemesia pallens* plant extract is subjected to analysis using GCMS and FTIR techniques. The Green-TiO_2 nanoparticles, doxorubicin drug loaded TiO_2 nanoparticles are characterized using several other techniques like XRD, FTIR, SEM, TEM, EDAX also.

5.3.1 GCMS

The GCMS analysis reveals that the major component found in extract are 5-hepten-3- one, 5, 5-Dimethyl-2(5H)- Furanone and 2-pentanol, along with other minor constituents and these are expected to be responsible for the hydrolysis of the precursor of TiO_2

5.3.2 FTIR

The Bio-Extract, Green-TiO_2, Green TiO_2–DoX nanoparticles and Doxorubicin drug are subjected to FTIR analysis. In Bio-Extract spectrum, peaks corresponding to free hydroxyl groups, asymmetric C-H stretching, aromatic ring, small ketonic group peak are observed. The FTIR spectrum of Green-TiO_2 nanoparticles showed metal oxide peak, plane bending vibrations peak of O-H and CO_2 molecules and the C-O-H bending band. The Green TiO_2-DoX spectrum contains peak corresponding to different quinine and ketone groups. The peaks due to primary amine NH_2 and N-H deformation bands and carbonyl group are found in both DoX spectrum and Green TiO_2-DoX spectrum. The peaks of Artemisia pallens spectrum is also seen in TiO_2-DoX spectrum. All these observations confirm the drug, DoX loaded into Green- TiO_2 nanoparticles. This suggests that the solvent has greater influence in the Green-TiO_2 nano carrier.

5.3.3 XRD

In XRD pattern of the Green-TiO_2 nanoparticles and Green-TiO_2-DoX have two prominent peaks observed at $2\theta=25.65°$, $48.37°$ and corresponds to (101), (200) reflection. The XRD of TiO_2 –DoX show extra peak at 31.5° corresponds to DoX. The crystallite size was calculated using Debye-Scherer equation and found to be 9-16nm.

5.3.4 UV-Vis spectrum

The UV absorption peak value of TiO_2 nanoparticles is 319 nm, The band gap is calculated and found to be 3.2 ev. Whereas the uv absorption peak value for DoX doped TiO_2 is shifted to 483 nm. This shift in UV peak confirms the doping of doxorubicin drug to TiO_2 nanoparticles.

5.3.5 SEM and TEM

The SEM images of Green-TiO_2 nanoparticle shows tetragonal shapes with different sizes. The Green-TiO_2 nano particles have relatively uniform structures with the mean particle range from 9-16nm with hexagonal shape as revealed from TEM. The Selective Area Diffraction pattern SAED was found to be in good agreement with the XRD observations. Both XRD and SAED patterns confirming the presence of Anatase phase in Green-TiO_2

5.3.6 MTT Assay

It was observed that reduction in cell viability using Green-TiO_2, DoX and Green-TiO_2-DoX, the experimental data reveals the fact that the increase in the concentration of drug carriers decreases the metabolic activity.

CONCLUSION

- *Artemisia pallen*, a native plant material can be used for the preparation of Bio-Ectract, a eco-friendly, bio-economic approach.
- Bio-Extracts were obtained using doubly-distilled water, a water boned and solvent free, eco-friendly approach.
- Naturally available flavanoids present in the Bio-Extract, such as 5,5-Dimethyl-2(5H)-Furanone and 2-Pentanol were effectively employed on solvent during the synthesis of TiO_2.

- We have successfully synthesized the TiO_2 using water-based Bio-Extract, as solvent for the hydrolysis and condensation reactions, a cleaner and greener approach.

- Bio-Extract based synthesized products, we label as Green-TiO_2 and found to be pure anatase phase, as revealed from XRD patterns.

- Band-Gap value of Green-TiO_2 obtained using Bio-Extract was found to be 3.2 as revealed from UV absorption spectrum.

- We obtained a particle size of Green-TiO_2 in the range of 9-16nm without any capping agent along with uniform hexagonal shapes, as revealed from SEM and TEM images.

- A successful effort was made to anchor a anti-cancer drug, DoX over Green-TiO_2 as its natural pH 6.0 for 6h equilibration time.

- Experimental results reveals that the drug, DoX encapsulated over Green-TiO_2 can be effectively employed as Nano Carrier for drug delivery systems.

- DoX laden Green-TiO_2, nano carrier was tested with human cervical cancer cell line, HeLa.

- Cyto toxicity of the Bio-Extract alone was tested through Cell viability analysis and the experimental result reveals good Cyto-compatibility towards HeLa cells upto 100µl/ml concentration with 98% cell viability.

- Effect of DoX on cell inhibition analysis reveals the fact that the cell inhibition was highly concentration dependent. The experimental data suggest that the rate of inhibition increased with increase in the concentration of DoX. Further, the IC 50 of free DoX against HeLa eas found to be 0.28.

- Effect of Green-TiO_2, nano carrier alone on HeLa cell viability was tested for 48h with different concentration of Green-TiO_2 the cell viability was found to be 99.12, 99.14, 94.29, 87.93 and 81.06% for 0.05. 0.50, 5.0, 50 and 100µg/ml of Green-TiO_2 respectively. This result suggests the bio-compatibility of Green-TiO_2 and can be used as a potential Nano carrier for drug delivery systems.

- In-Vitro toxicity of the concentration of Green-TiO_2-DoX on HeLa cell, the percent inhibition was found to be 1.24, 7.16, 22.00 and 34.28 for 0.5, 5.0, 50 and 100μg/ml, respectively.
- It is expected that, the drug, DoX released from the nano carrier, Green-TiO_2 in a time-dependent manner. This might have an added advantage that the time dependent drug release does not affect the normal cells through passive diffusion mechanism. The results also shows that as time increases the rate of drug release increases along with the increase in the concentration, consequently, inhibiting the cell growth in a time-dependent manner.

Suggestion for Future Research

- Based on our preliminary research on pure cell lines, animal studies will be carried out.
- The anti-tumor activity of DoX laden Green – TiO_2 will be activated by photo-induced electrons, called Photo Dynamic Therapy (PDT) with pure cell lines.
- Based on the current prelimary results and future PDT results, animal studies will be carried out.

References

Ahmad, A., Senapati, S., Khan, M.I., Kumar, R., Ramani, R., Srinivas, V., Sastry, M. (2003). "Intracellular synthesis of gold nanoparticles by a novel alkahol tolerant actinomycete Rhodococcus species". Nanotechnology.,14, 824–828.

Ahmad, A., Senapati, S., Khan, M.I., Kumar, R., Sastry M., (2003), "Extracellular biosynthesis of monodisperse goldnanoparticles by a novel extremophilicactinomycete, Thermomonospora sp". Langmuir., 19, 3550–3553.

Ahmad, A., Senapati, S., Khan, M.I., Kumar, R., Sastry M., (2005). "Extra-/intracellular, biosynthesis of goldnanoparticles by an alkalotolerant fungus, Trichothecium sp". J. Biomed. Nanotechnol., 1, 47–53.

Al-Salim, N.I., Bagshaw, S.A., Bittar, A., Kemmtt, T., Maquillan, A.J., Mills, A.M., and Ryan, M.J. (2000). Characterization and activity of sol-gel prepared TiO_2photocatalysts modified with Ca, Sr or Ba ion additives. J. Mater. Chem., 10: 2358-2363

Ambasta S P. (2000) Editor in Chief The Useful Plants of India. India: National Institute of Science and Communication (CSIR);

Aznar E., Climent E., Mondragon L., Sancenón F., Martínez-Máñez R.(2015)., "Functionalized Mesoporous Materials with Gate-Like Scaffoldings for Controlled Delivery. Polymers in Regenerative Medicine". Biomedical Applications from Nano-to Macro-Structures.,337–366.

Bali, R.R., N.; Lumb, A. & Harris, A.T. (2006). "The synthesis of metal nanoparticles inside liveplants".IEEE Xplore.

Baudhuin P., Vander Smisssen P., Beavois S., and Courtoy J.,(1989). "Molecular interactions between colloidal gold, protiens, and living cells in colloidal gold: Principles, Methods, and Applications", M.A.Hayat, Ed., 1-2, Academic press.

Baur V.W. H. (1961). "Atom and bindings with limnite brookite, TiO_2" ActaCrystallogr, 14: 214–216.

Beck-Broichsitter M., Merkel O.M., Kissel T. (2012). "Controlled pulmonary drug and gene delivery using polymeric nano-carriers". Journal of Controlled Release., 161:214–224.

Bernd, N. and Thomas, D.B. (2007). "Occurrence, behavior and effects of nanoparticles in the environment". Environ.Pollut., 150 (1): 5-22.

Bessekhouad Y., Robert D., and Weber J. V., (2003). "Preparation of TiO_2 nanoparticles by Sol-Gel route", International Journal of Photoenergy., 5(3):153-158

Boujday, S., Wunsch, F., Portes, P., Bocquet, J.F. and Justin, C.C. (2004). "Photo catalytic and electronic properties of TiO_2 powders elaborated by sol-gel route and supercritical drying". Solar Energy Mater. Solar Cells., 83(4): 421-433.

Buzea, C., Pacheco, I.I and Robbie, K. (2007). "Nanomaterials and Nanoparticles, Sources and toxicity". Biointerphases, 2(4): MR17-MR71.

Byun. D, Kim. Y, Lee. K, Hofmann. P., (2000). "Photocatalytic TiO_2 deposition by chemical vapor deposition" J.Haz. Mater.,73(2):199-206.

Carp O., Huisman C. L., Reller A.(2004). "Photoinduced reactivity of titanium dioxide". Prog in Solid State Chem., 32: 33–117.

Chadha T.S., Chattopadhyay S., Venkataraman C., Biswas P. (2012) "Study of the charge distribution on liposome particles aerosolized by air-jet atomization". Journal of aerosol medicine and pulmonary drug delivery., 25:355–364.

Chattopadhyay S. (2013). "Aerosol generation using nanometer liposome suspensions for pulmonary drug delivery applications". Journal of liposome research., 23:255–267.

Chaudhary A. (2011) "AyurvedicBhasma: nanomedicine of ancient India—its global contemporary perspective". Journal of biomedical nanotechnology., 7:68–69.

Che E., Gao Y., Wan. L, Zhang Y., Han N., Bai J., Li J., Sha Z., Wang S.(2015). "Paclitaxel/gelatin coated magnetic mesoporous silica nanoparticles: Preparation and antitumor efficacy in vivo. Microporous and Mesoporous". Materials., 204:226–234.

Chen X., Mao S.S. (2007.) "Titanium dioxide nano - materials: Synthesis, properties, modifications and applications". Chem. Rev., 107:2891–2959.

Chittasupho, C., Xie, S.X., Baoum, A., Yakovelva T., Siahaan, T.J., Berkland, C.J., (2009). "ICAM-1 targetting of doxorubicin-loaded PLGA nanoparticles to lung epithelial cells". Eur. J. Pharm. Sci., 37,141-150.

Chung C., Kim Y.K., Shin D., Ryoo S.R., Hong B.H., Min D.H. (2013) "Biomedical Applications of Graphene and Graphene Oxide". Accounts of Chemical Research., 46:2211–2224.

Corr, S.A. (2013). "Metal oxide nanoparticles" (Eds. O' Brien, P. and P. Paul), Nanoscience, The Royal Society of Chemistry, p. 180-207.

Csaba N., Garcia-Fuentes M., Alonso M.J., (2009). "Nanoparticles for nasal vaccination". Advanced Drug Delivery Reviews., 61:140–157.

DReyes-Coronado., G.Rodríguez-Gattorno, M.E.Espinosa Pesqueira, C. Cab, R.de Coss and G. Oskam, "Phase-pure TiO$_2$ nanoparticles: anatase, brookite and rutile" Nanotechnololgy., 19(14).

Dameron, C.T.; Reeser, R.N.; Mehra, R.K.; Kortan, A.R.; Carroll, P.J.; Steigerwald, M.L.; Brus, L.E.;Winge, (1989). "D.R. Biosynthesis of cadmium sulphide quantum semiconductor crystallites". Nature., 338,596–597.

Dames P., Gleich B., Flemmer A., Hajek K., Seidl N., Wiekhorst F., Eberbeck. D, Bittmann. I, Bergemann. C, Weyh T.(2007) "Targeted delivery of magnetic aerosol droplets to the lung". Nature nanotechnology., 2:495–499.

Das R.K., Gogoi N. and Bora U., (2011). "Green synthesis of gold nanoparticles using *Nyctanthes arbortristis* flower extract". Bioprocess Biosyst Eng., 34, 615-619

De Villiers, MM.;Aramwit, P.; Kwon, (2008.). "Nanotechnology in drug delivery". Springer Science & Business Media; 662

Dinwiddie R. (2005). "Anti-inflammatory therapy in cystic fibrosis. Journal of cystic fibrosis": Official journal of the European Cystic Fibrosis Society., 4:45–48.

Don T. Cromer and Herrington K., (1955). "The structures of anatase and rutile" J. Am. Chem. Soc., 77(18): 4708-4709.

Dubey S.P., Lahtinen M., Särkkä H. and Sillanpää M., (2010). "Bioprospective of *Sorbusaucuparia*leaf extract indevelopment of silver and gold nanocolloids". Colloids surf Biointerfaces., 80, 26-33.

Dusi, T., Mallat, A., Baiker, (1999), J of Molec Catal. A., Chem., 138,(1):15-23.

Dykman L., Khlebtsov N., (2012). "Gold nanoparticles in biomedical applications: recent advances and perspectives". Chemical Society Reviews., 41:2256–2282.

Farokhzad O.C., Langer R. (2009). "Impact of nanotechnology on drug delivery". ACS Nano., 3:16–20.

Fujishima A., Rao T.N., Tryk D.A. (2000). "Titanium dioxide photo catalysis". J Photochem Photobiol C Photo chem Rev., 1:1–21

G.M. Pajonk, (1991) "Aerogel Catalysts", Appl.Catal., 72(2):217-266.

G.Petrini, A.Cesana, G.deAlberti, F.Genoni, P.Rofia,(1991). Stud. Surf. Sci. Catal., 68:761-766.

Gao X., Wachs E., (1999) "Titania-Silica as catalysts: Molecular Structural Characteristics ad Physico-Chemical Properties", Catal. Today., 51(2):233-254.

Gelperina S., Kisich K., Iseman M.D., Heifets L. (2005). "The potential advantages of nanoparticle drug delivery systems in chemotherapy of tuberculosis. American journal of respiratory and critical care medicine., 172:1487–1490.

Gericke, M., Pinches, (2006), "A. Biological synthesis of metal nanoparticles". Hydrometallurgy., 83, 132–140.

Gillies,E.R., Frechet J.M.J.,(2005). "pH-responsive copolymer assemblies for controlled release of doxorubicin". Bioconjug. Chem.,16, 361-368.

H.C. Youn, S.Baral, J.H.Fendler, (1988.) "Preparations of nanosized TiO$_2$ in reverse micro emulsion," J. Phys.Chem. 92(22):6320-6327.

Hagerman J.K., Hancock K.E., Klepser M.E., (2006). "Aerosolised antibiotics: a critical appraisal of their use". 3:71–86.

Hay J.N., Raval H.M., (1998) "Solvent –free synthesis of binary inorganic oxides", J.Mater.Chem., 8(5):1233-1239.

Hench L.L. and West J.K., (1990) The Sol-gel-Process. Chemical Reviews,.90(1): 33-72

Hiremath S., Vidya C., Antonyraj M.A. L., Chandiaprabha M. N., Seemasshri S.(2014) "Green synthesis of TiO$_2$ nanoparticles by using neem leaf extract", Int. Rev.Appl. Bio. And biochem., 2(1):11-17.

Hu Y., Tsai H.L., Huang C.L., (2003), "Phase transformation of precipitated TiO$_2$ nanoparticles". Mater Sc Eng A., 344: 209–214

Hudlikar M., Joglekar S., Dhaygude M., Kodam K. (2012). "green synthesis of TiO$_2$ nanoparticles by using aqueous extract of jatrophacurcas L. latex", Mat. Lett., 75: 196-199.

Hughes G.A. (2005). "Nanostructure-mediated drug delivery. Nanomedicine": Nanotechnology, Biology and Medicine.; 1:22–30.

Hussain A., Virmani O.P., Sharma A., Kumar A., Misra L.N., Lucknow, India: (1998) Central Institute of Medicinal and Aromatic Plants;. Major Essential oil Bearing Plants of India.

Husseiny, M.I.; El-Aziz, M.A.; Badr, Y.; Mahmoud, M.A.(2007). "Biosynthesis of gold nanoparticles using Pseudomonas aeruginosa". Spectrochim.Acta A., 67, 1003–1006.

Jegadeeswaran P., Shivaraj R. and Venckatesh R., (2012). "Green synthesis of silver nanoparticles from extract of *Padinatetra stromatica* leaf". Dig J NanomaterBios., 7, 991-998.

Joerger, T.K.; Joerger, R.; Olsson, E.; Granqvist,(2001). "C.G. Bacteria as workers in the living factor: Metalaccumulating bacteria and their potential for materials science." Trends Biotechnol., 19, 1520.

Jung S., Patzelt A., Otberg N., Thiede G., Sterry W., Lademann J. (2009). "Strategy of topical vaccination with nanoparticles". Journal of biomedical optics. 14:021001–021007.

Kiyoshi Kanie and Tadao Sugimoto,(2004). "Shape control of anatase TiO_2 nanoparticles by amino acids in a gel–sol System", 1584-1585

Klein S., Weckhuysen B.M., Martens J.A, Majer W.F., Jacobs P.A., (1996) J.Catal 163,489-49.

Kowshik, M.; Arhtaputre, S.; Kharrazi, S.; Vogel,W.; Urban, J.; Kulkarni, S.K.; Paknikar, K.M. (2003). "Extracellular synthesis of silver nanoparticles by a silver-tolerant yeast strain MKY3". Nanotechnology, 14, 95–100.

Krishna, B. & Dan, V.G. (2009). "Silver nanoparticles for printable electronics and biological applications". J. Mater.Res., 24 (9): 2828-2836.

Kuber, C., Souza, S.F. (2006), "Extracellular biosynthesis of silver nanoparticles using the fungus Aspergillus fumigates". Colloids Surf. B., 47, 160–164.

Kumar T., Rahuman A.A., Jayaseelan C., Rajakumar G., Marimuthu S., Kirthi V.A., Velayutham K., Thomas J., Venkatesan., Kim K-S.(2014). "Green synthesis of titanium dioxide nanoparticles using *psidium guajava* extract and its antibacterial andantioxidant properties". Asian J Trop Med., pp. 968-976, doi: 10.1016/S1995-7645(14)60171-1.

Kumar, P.; Singh, P.; Kumari, K.; Mozumdar, S.; Chandra, R. (2011.) "A green approach for the synthesis of gold nano triangles using aqueous leaf extract of *Callistemon viminalis*". Mater.Lett., 65, 595–597.

Labhasetwar V. (2005). "Nanotechnology for drug and gene therapy: the importance of understanding molecular mechanisms of delivery". Current Opinion in Biotechnology.; 16:674–680.

Larsen, A.K., Escargueil, A.E., Sclandanowski, A. (2008), "Resistance mechanisms associated with altered intracellular distribution of anticancer agents". Pharmacol. Ther., 85, 217-229.

Latroche M., Brohan L., Marchand R, (1989.) "Newhollandite oxides: $TiO_2(H)$ and $K0.06TiO_2$". J Solid State Chem., 81: 78–82.

Lee W., Jeong M. C., and Young J. M. (2004), Nanotechnology., 15, 254.

Lee, S.W., Mao, C., Flynn, C., Belcher, A.M. (2002). "Ordering of quantum dots using genetically engineered viruses". Science, 296, 892–895

Lengke, M.; Southam, G. (2006). "Bioaccumulation of gold by sulphate-reducing bacteria cultured in the presence of gold (I)-thiosulfate complex". Acta., 70, 3646–3661.

Li Q.N., Wang X.M., Lu X.H., Tian H., Jiang H., Lv G,(2009). "The incorporation of Daunorubicin in cancer cells through the use of titanium dioxide whiskers". Biomaterials., 30: 4708–4715.

Li S., Shen Y., Xie A., Yu X., Zhang X., Yang L. and Li C., (2007). "Rapid, room-temperature synthesis of amorphous selenium protein composites using *Capsicum annuumL* extract". Nanotech.,18, (9).

Li, S.S., Y. Xie,A., Yu, X., Qui, L., Zhang, L., & Zhang, Q. (2007). "Green synthesis of silver nanoparticles using Capsicum annum L. extract". Green Chemistry., 9: 852-858.

Li, Y., White, T. J. and Lim, S.H. (2004). "Low temperature synthesis and micro structural control of titania nano particles". J. Sol. State Chem., 177(4-5): 1372-1381.

Liang X.J., Chen C., Zhao Y., Jia L, and Wang P.,(2008). "Biopharmaceutics and theraupetic potential of engineered nanomaterials". Current drug metabolism., 9(8): 697-709.

Linsebigler A.L, Lu G., Yates. J T. (1995). "Photo catalysis on TiO_2 surfaces: Principles, mechanisms, and selected results". Chem Rev., 95:735–758

Litter M. (1999). "Heterogenous photocatalysis transition metal ions in photocatalytic systems", Applied Catalysis B: Environmental., 23, 89-114.

Liu Z,. Davis R.J., (1994) "Investigation of the Structure of Micro porous Ti-Si Mixed Oxides by X-ray, UV Reflectance, Raman and FT-IR Spectroscopies", J. Phys.Chem., 98(4):1253-1261.

Lopez T., Sotelo J., Navarrete J., Ascencio J.A.(2006). "Synthesis of TiO_2 nanostructured reservoir with temozolomide: Structural evolution of the occluded drug". Optical Materials., 29: 88-94.

Marimuthu S., Rahuman A.A., Jayaseelan C., Kirthi V.A., Santoshkumar T., Velayutham K., Bagavan A., Kamraj C., Elango G., Iyappan M., Siva C., KarthikL., Rao B.V.K. (2013) "Acaricidal activity of synthesized titanium dioxide nano particles using *Calotropis gigantea* against rhipice phalusmicroplus and haemaphysalis bispinosa", Asian Paci. J. Trop. Med. 682-688.

Mari. B, Mollar. M, Mechkour. A, Hartiti. B, Perales. M, Cembrero. J, Microelectron. J., (2004), 35, 79.

Maynard, A.D. (2006). "Nanotechnology: A Research Strategy for Addressing Risk". Woodrow Wilson International Center for Scholars, Washington, DC.

McNeil, S.E. (2005). "Nanotechnology for the biologist". J. Leukoc. Biol., 78, 585-594.

Merzlyak, A.; Lee, S.W. (2006). "Phage as template for hybrid materials and mediators for nanomaterials synthesis Curr. Opin". Chem. Biol., 10, 246–252.

Mo S, Ching W. (1995). "Electronic and optical properties of three phases of titanium dioxide: Rutile, anatase and brookite". Phys Rev B., 51:13023–13032.

Mohamed S. Hamdy., (2014). "One step synthesis of M-Doped TiO_2 nanoparticles in TUD-1(M-TiO_2-TUD-1, M=Cr or V) and their photocatalytic performance under visible light radiation". Journal of Molecular catalysis A: Chemical., 39339-46.

Mohammed Ghanbari, Asadollah Asadi and Somayyeh Rostamzadeh., (2016). "Study of the Cytotoxicity effect of Doxorubicin- loaded/ Folic acid-Targeted Super Paramagnetic Iron Oxide Nanoparticles on AGS Cancer Cell Line". Journal of Nanomedicine & Nanotechnology., 7(2): 1000368

Mohanpuria,P.R., K.N. & Yadav,S.K,. "Biosynthesis of nanoparticles: technological concepts and future applications". Journal of Nanoparticle Research.10:507- 517.

Monticone, S., Tufeu, R., Kanaev, A.V., Scolan, E. and Sanchez, C. (2000). "Quantum size effect in TiO$_2$ nanoparticles: does it exist?" Appl.Surf.Sci., 162-163: 565-570

Mor G.K, Varghese O.K, Paulose M., (2006). "A review on highly ordered, Vertically oriented TiO$_2$ nanotube arrays: Fabrication, materialproperties, and solar energy applications". Solar Energy Mater Solar Cell., 90: 2011–2075

Motasim Bellah, Md., Shawn M. Christensen and Samir M. Iqbal (2011). Review article: Nanostructures for Medical Diagnostics. Journal of Nanomaterials, Volume 2012, Article ID 486301, 21 pages.

Mukherjee, P., Ahmad, A., Mandal, D., Senapati, S., Sainkar, S.R., Khan, M.I., Parishcha, R., Aiayumar, P.V., Alam, M., Kumar, R., (2001). "Fungus-mediated synthesis of silver nanoparticles and their immobilization inthe mycelia matrix: A novel biological approach to nanoparticles synthesis". Nano Lett., 1, 515–519.

Muscat J., Swamy V., Harrison N.M.(2002), "First-principles calculations of the phase stability of TiO$_2$ ". Phy Rev B., 65: 1–15.

Nair, B., Pradeep, T. (2002). "Coalescence of nanoclusters and formation of submicron crystallites assisted byLactobacillus strains". Cryst. Growth Des., 2, 293–298.

Nel, A., Xia. T., Madler, L., and Li, N. (2006). "Toxic potential of materials at the nanolevel". Science., 311, 622-627.

Nithya A., Rokesh K., Jothivenkatachalam K.(2013). "biosynthesis, characterizationand application of titanium dioxide nanoparticles", Nano vision., 3(3): 169-174.

Njagi C.E., Huang H., Stafford L., Genuino H., GalindoM.H., Collins B.J., Hoag E.G. and Suib L.S., (2011). "Biosynthesisof iron and silver nanoparticles at room temperature usingaqueous *Sorghum* bran extracts". Langmuir.,27, 264-271

Norotsky A., Jamieson J.C, Kleppa O.J. (1967). "Enthalpy of transformation of a high pressure polymorph of titanium dioxide to the rutile modification". Science., 158: 338–389.

O'Riordan T.G. (2005); "Aerosol delivery devices and obstructive airway disease". 2:197–203.

Pal D., Sahu C.K, Haldar A. Bhasma. (2014). "The ancient Indian nanomedicine". Journal of advanced pharmaceutical technology & research., 5:4–12.

Parashar, U.K.S., S.P. & Srivastava, A., "Bioinspired synthesis of silver nanoparticles". (2009). Digest journal Of nanomaterials and biostructures., 4(1):159- 166.

Park. H and Park J. G., (2006). "Synthesis of Ultrawide ZnO Nanosheets,". Curr. Appl.Phys., 6, 1020–3

Philip, D. (2010). "Green synthesis of gold and silver nanoparticles using Hibiscus rosasinensis". Phys. E, 42,1417–1424.

Pridgen E.M, Alexis F., Farokhzad O.C. (2015). "Polymeric nanoparticle drug delivery technologies for oral delivery applications. Expert opinion on drug delivery". 1–15.

Rajakumar G., Rahuman A.A., Priyamvada B., Khanna V.G., Kumar D.K., Sujin P.J.(2012). "Eclipta prostrate leaf aqueous extract mediated synthesis of titanium dioxide nanoparticles", Mat. Lett., 68:115-117.

Ramgir N. S., Late D. J., Bhite A. B., More M. A., Mulla I. S. Joag D. S., and K. Vijayamohanan, (2006), J. Phys. Chem. B., 110, 18236.

Ramimoghadam D., Bagheri S., Hamid A.S.B.(2014). "Biotemplated synthesis of anatase titanium dioxide nanoparticles via lingo cellulosic waste material", Biomed. Res.Int.,205636, 1-7.

Rao G.K., Ashok C., RaoV.K., Chakra S.C., Rajendar V.(2015). "Synthesis of TiO_2 nanoparticles from orange fruit waste", Int. J. Multidis. Adv. Res. Tren., 2(1): 82-90.

Rao R., Markovic S., Anderson P. (2003). "Aerosol therapy for malignancy involving the lungs". Current cancer drug targets. 3:239–250.

Raveendran, P.F., J. &Wallen., S.L., (2003). Completely ""Green" Synthesis and Stabilization of metal nanoparticles". Journal of American Chemical Society., 125(46):13940-13941.

Rodriguez-Sanchez, L., Blanco, M.C. & Lopez-Quintela, M.A., (2000). "Electrochemical synthesis of silver nanoparticles". J. Phys. Chem. B., 104 (41): 9683-9688.

Roh, Y., Lauf, R.J., McMillan, A.D., Zhang, C., Rawn, C.J., Bai, J., Phelps, T.J. (2001). "Microbial synthesis and the characterization of metal-substituted magnetites". Solid State Commun., 118, 529–534.

Roopan S.M, Bharathi A., Prabhakaran A., Rahuman A.A, Velayutham K, Rajakumar G.,(2012). "Efficient phyto-synthesis and structural characterization of rutile TiO_2 nanoparticles using Annonasquamosa peel extract". A Mol Biomol Spectrosc; 98: 86-90.

Rosi N.L. and Mirkin C.A.,(2005). "Nanostructures in biodiagnostics" Chemical reviews., 105(4):1547-1562.

Ruiz, A.M., Sakai, G., Cornet, A., Shimanoe, K., Morante, J.R. and Yamazoe, N. (2004). "Microstructure control of thermally stable TiO_2 obtained by hydrothermal process for gas sensors". Sens. Actuators B: Chem., 103(1-2): 312-317.

S. Baker and K. S. K. P. S. akshith, (2013). "Plants: Emerging as nanofactories towards facile route in synthesis of nanoparticles," BioImpacts., 3(3): 111-117.

Sahoo S.K., Labhasetwar V. (2003). "Nanotech approaches to drug delivery and imaging". Drug discovery today. 8:1112–1120.

Salam H.A., Sivaraj R.(2014) "OcimumbasilicumL. var. purpurascens Benth.- lamiaceae mediated green synthesis and characterization of titanium dioxide nanoparticles", Advances in Biores.,5(3): 10-16.

Sastry, M.; Ahmad, A.; Khan, M.I.; Kumar, R. (2003). "Biosynthesis of metal nanoparticles using fungi andactinomycete". Curr. Sci., 85, 162–170.

Saxena, A., Tripathi, R.M. & Singh, R.P. (2010). "Biological synthesis of silver nanoparticles using onion (*Alliumcepa*) extract and their antibacterial activity". Dig. J. Nanomater. Biostruc., 5 (2): 427-432.

Schraml-Marth M., Walther K.L., Wokaun A.,(1992). "Porous silica gels and TiO_2/SiO_2 mixed oxides", J. Non-Cryst. Solids.,143:93-111.

Sclafani A., Palmisano L., Schiavello M. (1990). "Influence of the preparation methods of titanium dioxide on the photocatalytic degradation of phenol in aqueous dispersion". J PhysChem., 94: 829–832.

Selloni A. (2008). "Anatase shows its reactive side". Nature Mater., 7:613–615.

Senthilkumaar S., Porkodi K., Gomathi R., Geetha M.A., Manonmani N. "Sol–gel derived silver doped nanocrystalline titania catalysed photo degradation of methylene blue from aqueous solution". Dyes Pigm., 2006; 69: 22-30.

Sergio Valencia, Ximena Vargas, Luis Rios, Gloria Restrepo, Juan M, Marin. (2013). "Sol-Gel and low-temperature solvothermal synthesis of photoactive nano-titanium dioxide". Journal of Photochemistry and Photobiology A: Chemistry., 251(2013)175-181.

Shafiu Abdhulla Kamba, Maznah Ismail, Samer Hasan Hussein-Al-Ali, Tengku Azmi Tengku Ibrahim and Zuki Abu Bakar Zakaria., (201b3,) *In Vitro* Delivery and Controlled Release of Doxorubicin for Targeting Osteosarcoma Bone Cancer" Molecules., 18, 10580-10598.

SharmilaDevi R., Venckatesh Dr.R, Dr.Rajeshwari Sivaraj, (2014) "Synthesis of Titanium Dioxide Nanoparticles by Sol-Gel Technique" IJIRSET., 3(8).

Shi, H., Magaye, R., Castranova, V., and Zhao, J., (2013). "Titanium dioxide nanoparticles: a review of current toxicological data. Part". Fibre Toxicol., 10(4): 1-33.

Singh A., Jain D., Upadhyay M.K., Khandelwal N. andVerma H.N., (2010). "Green synthesis of silver nanoparticles using *Argemone mexicana* leaf extract and evaluation of their antimicrobial activities". Dig J NanomaterBios., 5, 483-489

Singh P.R., Shukla K.V., Yadav S.R., Sharma K.P., SinghK.P. and Pandey C.A., (2011). "Biological approach of zinc oxide nanoparticles formation and its characterization. Adv. Mat.Lett., 2, 313-317

Simons P.Y., and Dachille F. (1967). "The structure of TiO_2 II, a high pressure phase of TiO_2". Acta Crystallographica., 23:334.

Smith J.D., Morton L.D., Ulery B.D. (2015), "Nanoparticles as synthetic vaccines". Current opinion in biotechnology., 34:217–224.

Song J.Y., Kwon E.Y. and Kim B.S., (2010). "Biological synthesisof platinum nanoparticles using *Diopyros kaki* leaf extract". Bioprocess Biosyst Eng., 33, 159–164

Song J. H, Wang X. D, Riedo. E, and Wang Z. L. (2005). "Elastic property of vertically aligned nanowires". J. Phys. Chem. B., 109: 9869-9872.

Sotelo. J.L. VanGrieken R., Martos, C. (1999). "Catalytic aerogel-like materials dried at ambient pressure for liquid-phase epoxidation", ChemCommun., 6:549-550.

Subhashini D., Nachiyar C.V. (2014). "Albiziasaman: a green route for the reduction of bulk TiO_2", Int. J. Chem Tech Res., 6(12): 5137-5141.

Sundrarajan M., and Gowri S. (2011). "Green synthesis of titaniumdioxide nanoparticles by *Nyctanthes arbor-tristis* leaves extract. Chalcogenidelet., 8, 447- 451

Taleb, A., Petit, C. & Pileni, M.P.(1997). "Syntheses of highly mono disperse silver nanoparticles from AOT reverse micelles: a way to 2D and 3D self-organization". Chem. Mater., 9 (4): 950-959.

Tanaka K., Capule M.F. V, Hisanaga T. (1991). "Effect of crystallinity of TiO_2 on its photocatalytic action". ChemPhysLett., 187: 73–76.

Thirunavukkarasu Santhoshkumar, Abdul Abdul Rahuman, Chidambaram Jayaseelan, Govindasamy Rajakumar, Sampath Marimuthu, Arivarasan Vishnu Kirthi, KanayairamVelayutham, John Thomas, Jayachandran Venkatesan, Se- Kwon Kim. (2014). "Green synthesis of titanium dioxide nanoparticles using *Psidiumguajava*extract and its antibacterial and antioxidant properties". Asian Pacific Journal of Tropical Medicine 968-976.

Thompson T L, Yates J. T (2006). "Surface science studies of the photo activation of TiO_2-New photochemical processes". Chem Rev., 106: 4428–4453.

Toba M., Mizukami F., Niwa S., Sano T., Maeda K., Annila A., Komppa V, (1994). "Effect of the type of preparation the properties of Titania/Silicas", J.Molec.Catal., 91(2): 277-289,.

Torresday, J.L.G.P., Gomez, E.; Videa, J.P.; Troiani, H.E.; Santiago, P. & Yacaman, M.J. (2002). "Formation and growth of Au nanoparticles inside live alfaalfa plants". Nanoletters, 2(4): 397- 401.

Tripathi, R.M., Saxena, A., Gupta, N., Kapoor, H. & Singh, R.P. (2010). High antibacterial activity of silver nanoballs against *E. coli* MTCC 1302, *S. typhimurium* MTCC 1254, *B. subtilis* MTCC 1133 and *P. aeruginosa* MTCC 2295". Dig.J. Nanomater. Biostruc., 5 (2): 323-330.

Valli G. Geetha S. (2015). "A green method for the synthesis of titanium dioxide nanoparticles using cassia auriculata leaves extract", Euro. J. Biomed. Phar Sci., 2(3): 490-497.

Vayssieres, L. Keis K., Lindquist S. E., (2001), A. Hagfeldt, J. Phys. Chem. B., 105, 3350.

Velayutham K., Rahuman. A.A., Rajakumar G., Marimuthu S., Santhoshkumar. T, Jayaseelan. C, (2011), "Evaluation of Catharanthus roseus leaf extract-mediated biosynthesis of titanium dioxide nanoparticles against Hippobosca maculate and Bovicolaovis". Parasitol Res; 111(6): 2329-2337.

Venkatachalam N., Palanichamy M., Murugesan V.,(2007). "Sol–gel preparation and characterization of nanosize TiO_2: Its photocatalytic performance", Materials Chemistry and Physics., 104,454–459

Wagner R. S. and Ellis W. C., (1964), Appl. Phys. Lett., 4, 89.

Wang X. D., Song J. H., Li P. Ryon J. H., Dupu R. D., Summers C. J., and.Wang Z. L. (2005), J. Am. Chem. Soc., 127, 7920.

Wang X. D., Summers C. J., and Wang Z. L., Nano. Lett., 4, 423.

Ward D.A, Ko.E.I (1995) "Preparing Catalytic Materials by the Sol-Gel Method", Chem. Res., 34(2):421-433.

Wenzhi Ren, Leyong Zeng, Zheyu Shen, Lingchao Xiang, An Gong, Jichao Zhang, Chengwen Mao, Aiguo Li, Tatjana Panuesku, Gayle E. Woloschak, Narayan S, Hosmane and Aiguo Wu., (2013), "Enhanced doxorubicin transport to multidrug resistant breast cancer cells via TiO_2 nanocarriers". RSC Advances., 3,20855

Wright J.D and Sommerdijk N.A.J.M., Sol-gel-Materials: Chemistry and applications. Advanced Chemistry Texts.2001: Gordon and Breach Science Publishers.

Yang P. D., Yan H., Mao S., Russo R., Johnson J., Saykally R., Morris N., Adv. Funct. Mater., (2002), 12, 323.

Yi K.C., Fendler J.H., (1990) "Between the Head groups of Langmuir-Blodgett Films", Langmuir., 6(9):1519-1521.

Yin Z.F., Wu L., Yang H.G., Su Y.H. (2013). "Recent progress in biomedical applications of titanium dioxide". Phys Chem., 15: 4844-4858.

You X., Chen F, Zhang J.(2005). "Effects of calcination on the physical and photocatalytic properties of TiO_2 powders prepared by sol-gel template method". J Sol-Gel Sci Tech, 34: 181–187.

Zhang Q, Gao L, Guo J.(2000). "Effects of calcination on the photocatalytic properties of nanosized TiO_2 powders prepared by TiCl4 hydrolysis". ApplCatal B Environ, 26: 207–215.

Zhao Q. X., Klason P., and Willander M., (2007), Appl. Phys.A., 88, 27.

ABOUT THE AUTHORS

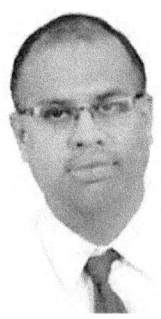

Dr. S. Senthilkumaar, presently working as Assistant Professor – Senior Grade in the Department of Chemistry, PSG College of Technology, Coimbatore, Tamil Nadu since 2001. He has 21 years of total teaching, research and industrial experience. He was the recipient of "Young Scientist Award" offered by the Tamil Nadu State Council for Science and Technology in the year 2003. His areas of research interest are Nano Catalysts for Organic reactions, non-toxic agricultural biomass for Environmental Remediation, Environmental Photochemistry, Ceramics, composite materials, inorganic ion-exchangers for detoxicification of ground water and Nano Carriers for drug delivery for malignant cells. To his credit, he has published more than 50 research articles in an international peer-reviewed journals published from ACS, IOP, Elsevier, etc. He is honored by Editors of several journals published from Elsevier, John Wiley, ACS by appointing him as a regular reviewer for their journals, as a token of his contribution. He has very good citation index. He has produced 7 PhD students under his guidance as on 2016. Most of his full-time research students are the recipient of National Doctoral Research Fellowship offered by AICTE, New Delhi. He delivered key note address in several national and international conferences and also served as a session chairman. He is also serving as a Board of Studies member in many of the autonomous Engineering College under Anna University and Arts and Science College under Bharathiar University.

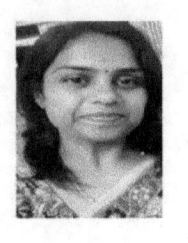

M. Mythreyi has done her Masters in Environmental Science in Anna University, Chennai and currently has submitted her PhD thesis in Environmental Sciences in PSG College of Arts and Science Coimbatore. Also is a IEMA certified Lead Auditor for Environmental Management Systems and currently practicing as a consultant for EMS, OSHAS and Food Safety Audits.

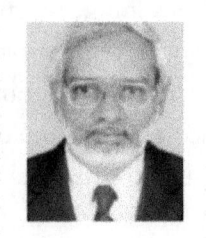

Dr. S. Pattabhi is a Active researcher and Able administrator. He headed the department of Environmental Sciences PSG college of arts and science for more than three decades. He is known for his outstanding research contribution in the field of Waste Water Treatment, Bio-Methanization and Cost-effective adsorbent development. He has more than 80 peer reviewed research publications with high impact factor.

www.ingramcontent.com/pod-product-compliance
Lightning Source LLC
Chambersburg PA
CBHW051728170526
45167CB00002B/843